TURNING WHITE
A Memoir of Change

FEB 08

TURNING WHITE
A Memoir of Change

Lee Thomas

Published by Momentum Books, L.L.C.

2145 Crooks Road, Suite 208
Troy, Michigan 48084
www.momentumbooks.com
Printed in Canada

ISBN-13: 978-1-879094-81-9
ISBN-10: 1-879094-81-9
LCCN: 2007936661

Cover photographs by Michael Shore

To Ethel Lois,
When I think of you my heart swells,
and words escape me except for one: "Love."
Mom, thank you.

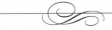

Contents

Foreword

I wonder what they see.

They squint for a split-second, then glance away when they realize I'm looking back at them. For those who dare to stare, their eyes widen with what can only be called shock … then it slowly turns to wrinkled-brow confusion. Then they look away. Others look at me with a shocked stare that persists until they realize I am actually looking back at them. Then they quickly step aside if they're walking toward me. The very old and the very young are especially guilty of the long stare.

Being noticed is something to which I've become accustomed, having been on television all of my adult life. It seems people are excited to see their local TV personality in person. But all stares are not the same. Even people who have known me for years avoid eye contact when they see my face without makeup for the first time.

In my head, I know that curiosity motivates the stares and weird responses. But this rational understanding doesn't always stop the emotion of the moment. These strangers and acquaintances are so distracted by what they see it seems like they do not realize that there is a man beneath the skin. They only see the drastic two-tones of my face as their eyes flash a thousand questions and a barrage of emotions that, at times, can be as unbearably awkward for them as it is for me.

But I confess, even I am awestruck by what is happening to my body. And that compels me to wrap words around all these emotions and try to share them. I am also sharing pictures of my ever-changing skin so people can see beyond my face and hands—how this disease is transforming the largest organ of my body.

It began with tiny seeds of whiteness, mysteriously sprinkled onto my brown skin, that suddenly sprouted into small circles. With ravenous, ruthless hunger, these discs of discoloration devoured every drop of pigment along their smooth and scalloped edges. The whiteness blossomed across my torso ... my nose ... my lips. It twined around my hands and feet, weaving pale gloves and boots in its wake.

Years later, these white splashes in my sea of brown skin have produced a phenomenon that I have devoted a good portion of my life to understanding and resolving in as many ways as possible. The photographs show these incredible contrasts of my skin, because I want people to see the body as human artwork, a compelling canvas that I am unveiling to the world.

These incredible pictures of a black man turning white used to shock me.

Now I am fascinated.

And eager to explain.

No, it's not a burn, even though it can leave an emotional sting. I have thought about telling people that my skin is this way because of a war injury that I suffered while defusing a bomb in Baghdad. But I'm a talker, not a fighter. Plus, my brother fought in the wars of this nation and I would never besmirch our military men and women, nor my family, with a self-serving lie.

The truth of the matter is simple and unflattering. The white that you see on this black man just appeared one day. I thought nothing of it, when out of the blue a single spot of white just appeared on my scalp. I had no idea that one seemingly insignificant blotch would irreversibly change my life in so many unbelievable ways.

Wait, sometimes I get ahead of myself. Let's start, my friends, with what these sprinkles of white are ... besides shocking. This is a disease called vitiligo. It's pronounced vit-ill-EYE-go. Now, hold on to your brainpan because here's the medical definition: Vitiligo is a pigmentation disorder in which the cells that make pigment, or melanocytes, in the skin and the mucous membranes—which are the tissues that line the inside of the mouth and nose as well as the genital and rectal area—are destroyed.

As a result, white patches appear on the skin across different parts of the body. Plus, the hair that grows in those affected areas turns white. OK, I know that's a mouthful—or should I say an eyeful. Simply put, it's more than turning white. It's becoming void of color. And it affects every ethnicity and skin color. But, of course, on darker skin it's a lot more noticeable.

My introduction to this disease was jarring and somewhat insensitive.

For nearly fifteen years, this skin disorder has transformed my color and my life and has given me a unique perspective on a very famous person whom I've never met. Because I understand one thing about the man better than most people. Michael Jackson is the greatest musical entertainer on the planet, and I'm sure he has some issues. But bleaching isn't one of them. Michael has vitiligo, the same disease that

I have. It's funny because it started on my scalp, then on one hand, then the other hand, and so on.

Remember when Michael used to wear one glove and it became a fashion statement? I bet he even had to laugh about that, because the man was probably covering up his spotted hand. Then when it advanced to both hands, he wore two gloves … and *that* wasn't such a fashion statement.

Anyway, I can confirm that bleaching is one of the recommended treatments if you have the disease over eighty percent of your body. He tried to explain that to Oprah Winfrey in the '90s and to a British journalist this decade. People didn't really believe him back then, plus there were so many other controversial things to talk about pertaining to Mr. Jackson. The British journalist didn't focus on that at all. He wasn't really wanting to hear about it. But if it means anything for the record, I vouch for Mr. Jackson when it comes the vitiligo.

I can say without question that this disease has given me moments of despair and has lifted me into amazingly euphoric epiphanies. It's kept me locked behind closed doors and sent me out to shout into the biggest microphone I can find. It has altered my outlook on life in profound ways. For that reason, I am sharing my story. I am doing this for myself and the many people who are living with this disease. According to the National Vitiligo Foundation, one to two percent of the population of the United States has this disease—that's two to four million Americans. I believe there are more … lots of people keeping their suffering a secret.

These men, women, and children are living their lives trying to follow their dreams and desires with an uncompromising enemy that looms like a shadow over everything in their world. Some choose to hide. I understand their struggles and pain. There is no cure. There are only treatments and theories about genetic causes for this autoimmune disorder. In my case, no one in my family as far back as my mother's grandfather has ever seen this disease. I hope my story can help answer the questions dancing in strangers' eyes and explain this skin-changing phenomenon, while at the same time help other people with vitiligo feel understood and accepted.

Thank you for reading my story.

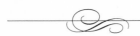

ONE

There Is No Cure

"YOU HAVE A DISEASE CALLED VITILIGO," the doctor said with a straight, no-chaser delivery that made the words sting even more brutally. This was New York City in 1994, during my second chance at a career in The Big Apple.

"It's where your skin just turns white for no reason. There is no cure."

As he continued speaking, the doctor's voice became the unintelligible drone of Charlie Brown's teacher. He was shuffling through papers on his desk, I think. I really didn't hear anything after he said, "There is no cure ... "

Those words echoed in my head for the next few minutes. The room seemed like a great chasm, humming with static.

But this room could not have felt as hollow as my stomach. My vision blurred as my gaze drifted toward the light. "No cure" muted and dimmed my world. My mouth gaped. At least, I *think* my mouth was open as I stared at the doctor. The shock of his words seemed to paralyze and numb me all at once. How could those two little white spots on my scalp, and the one forming on my hand, result in this horrific prognosis—"No cure!"

After torturously long moments of echoing, I focused on the doctor. The dude was still talking while I had reeled into limbo land. He was fussing with papers on his desk while his expression bore the frustration of someone who'd been repeating himself. His voice slowly transformed from the babble of Charlie Brown's teacher back to my doctor speaking plain English. I forced myself to listen. Somehow I regained control of my mouth.

"What's that, Doc?"

"We have treatments," he said.

"OK," I said, snapping back to coherence. "Back up for a second. There is no cure. I have spots on my head and hand. It turns white for no reason. There's no cure, but you have treatments."

The dermatologist just wasn't making sense. It was not jiving. They don't know the cause or the cure, but there are treatments. Rage and confusion exploded inside me. My emotions burst into an accusatory shout: "You're a doctor! You're supposed to know stuff!"

That's it. That's how the story begins. That awful, confusing doctor's visit launched me on a journey that has stretched around the globe for more than a decade and a half. It has propelled me to research, study, and consult with a multitude of experts in many countries. In person and by phone, I have put my journalistic skills to work on the most vexing, perplexing story of my life: How and where can I find a cure to this disease that is making me turn white?

Concrete answers to that question continue to elude me, just as they did that day in the New York dermatologist's office.

"This disease is not contagious or life-threatening," he told me. "Plus, there is not a lot of research in this area. And even though we don't know the cause, most people respond to the treatment."

He gave me a tube of cream that was supposed to stimulate the growth of brown pigment in my skin. Grasping that little tube was like physically grabbing onto a glimmer of hope.

"But there are also some who don't respond to treatment." The doctor's somber tone smashed my hope to bits. "For them, the disease takes over and they lose all pigment."

It still didn't make sense. "So if you don't know the cause, and you just treat the result," I asked, "won't it just come back?"

"That's possible."

And that's all he had to say. "That's possible." So I left the doctor's office that day—a black man turning white—with little hope of full recovery. I had only the possibility of "treatments" for a disease that has no cure.

Perfect, let's go be on TV.

Black Man Turning White, Live At Five

Seriously.

While news of this disease would devastate anyone, it was especially terrifying for me.

Let me explain what I do for a living. My job and my life-long dream were one and the same. Because after a lot of hard work, and even a few tears, my star was shining over the pinnacle of my profession. I was in a position that masses of people in my field would describe as being at the top. And I was loving it.

I was a feature/entertainment reporter for WABC-TV, the flagship station of the American Broadcasting Company—you know, ABC in New York City. My desk had once been the workspace of Rolanda Watts. She had her own nationally syndicated talk show in the '90s for four seasons before heading to Los Angeles for the life of an actor.

And here I was: heir to the throne. Here I was: a rising star in the super-competitive arena of broadcast journalism, in the top media market in the country, working in what many people describe as the communications capital of the planet. This was the job I had dreamed about since I was a little kid growing up in Oklahoma.

I vividly remember the day when the dream took hold of my young mind, flashing in Technicolor brilliance. The dream began with a commercial that featured a young actor named Rodney Allen Rippy, which I watched on the only television that our family owned.

We were all watching. "We" includes my three brothers, two sisters and myself, the baby. Right then and there, watching little Mr. Rippy, I knew what I wanted. All of five years old, I stood up between my siblings and the television.

"I can do that!" I proclaimed. "I want to be on TV!"

That was it. I had sent the dream soaring into the universe. All I had to do was grow up and make it happen. Just in case it didn't, I had a Plan B: We would front a family band like those Jacksons. But since my siblings didn't go for the singing thing, TV seemed like the right choice.

Now that I said it out loud, my dream was real. My

family's reply was supportive and somehow directly honest at the same time: "Of course you can," they said. "Just do it somewhere else. You're blocking the TV!"

I stood my ground, making sure they understood how serious I was about my newfound career.

"I can do that," I declared again. "I wanna be on TV."

Once the pillow hit my head, I knew it was time to move from in front of the tube. But the seed was planted. And it would take more than a multicolored couch pillow to knock it out of my brain.

So twenty years later when that doctor gave his callous diagnosis and condemned me with the words "no cure," he didn't just tell me that I was turning white. The translation meant much more. He was turning off the TV and sending me to bed forever. He was telling me the dream was over. And I would much rather be hit in the head with a pillow than in the gut with reality.

Crestfallen Star

After the doctor's appointment, I headed back to the TV station. Walking the bustling streets of Manhattan, my mind spun in a million directions, trying to make sense of what was happening.

I was twenty-five years old, working in New York City in

my chosen profession. This was a career that I had worked very hard to create and maintain. Yet my body was not cooperating with the dream—it was betraying me, threatening to change my appearance drastically.

"No cure!" The doctor's words gonged in my head as I made a detour into Central Park to think.

"I'm turning white," I told myself. I strode past joggers and bikers and mothers pushing baby carriages on the wooded paths in the middle of a city where my face beamed over the TV airwaves every day.

Hopelessness weighed heavily on my mind and body as I walked. There was no way for me to stop what was happening to my skin.

I didn't know what to do. Should I let the disease progress and allow my nightmare to be broadcast to the seventeen million or so viewers of the New York City metropolitan area? They could all tune in and watch the incredible black/white reporter turn colors with each broadcast.

Would a reporter who's turning white get booted off the TV screen? Did the millions of people who watched my reports every day want to see me change colors before their eyes? Would they be so distracted by my transformation that they would not pay attention to my interviews with movie stars or reports about the latest films?

I contemplated another option: I could just leave and go turn white all by myself on some island. I would be the guy in the multi-colored orange, brown, and yellow shirt, belly up to the bar every night, except weekends because I wouldn't be able to afford the drinks on those nights. But I would be able to dazzle the tourists on my island with my portable DVD player and copies of my old news reports at the ready. I would talk of past glory and impress the girls with my vast knowledge of television.

"What, I know that anchorman," I'd say with an all-knowing laugh. "He's a great guy. He and I used to be on the same newscast."

I would be just like a former high school football player, always reliving his glory days to relieve the pain of being a fallen star. But instead of a jersey, I would have a faded red tie and a newsboy cap with a coffee-stained press pass stapled to the front.

Damn, man! I thought the diagnosis meant I was going to have to give up my life.

Royal Celebrities

We live in a TV nation. This is a country where talk around the proverbial water cooler is the same as generations past, with one big difference:

"I can't believe she's sleeping with him. Well, everyone knew he was married when they met."

"You know, she's at least twenty-two years younger than him, plus I think he's a little crazy."

And they are not talking about the guy in the office down the hall. They are not referring to the next-door neighbor. It's all about American royalty.

They are referring to Hollywood celebrities. People all over this great country thrive on gossip. It's our common conversation. We all talk on a regular basis about people we don't even know:

"I can't believe Brad left Jen for Angelina ... but they make such a great couple."

It's fun.

"I can't believe that anchorman is black. I heard he turned white."

This is a nation in which the slightest change in a television personality's hairdo can be the topic of morning drive radio.

So, do you think a black man turning white on TV would go unnoticed?

As I walked down 67th Street from Central Park back to work, my mind was racing with reasons and scenarios that would herald the demise of my dream. In the lobby, I passed a picture of Regis Philbin and Kathy Lee Gifford. On the elevator up to the newsroom, I just happened to share the ride with Michael Gelman, Regis' friend and producer.

It was one of those epiphany moments that make you reflect and realize where you are, how you got there ... and just how phenomenal it really is.

Man, I was right in the middle of my dream coming true. I paid my way through college, making sure I got the education I would need to succeed in my chosen profession, only to lose the game because of a disease.

Come on, give me a break! Can I please just get some ailment that people can't see? But no-o-o-o, I have to go and start turning white. Unless this is going to help my credit report, I don't want it!

For the rest of the elevator ride, and the rest of the week for that matter, I cursed. I kicked. I screamed a barrage of "What the hell!" and "Why me?" You know, the typical stuff that destroyed dreams are made of. From everything that I could calculate, my fate was sealed. Because in this vapid world of television, a spotted black man equals unemployment.

The End Marks the Beginning

That is where this journey begins. I thought my career was over before I really even got it started.

Fortunately, I was wrong. As a matter of fact, I couldn't

have been more wrong. This would not be the first time I would be completely incorrect. It was, however, the first time I began to fight for something other than my career aspirations.

When I first thought of writing a book, it was going to be all about the cure for vitiligo. I was wrong about that as well, because it's turned into so much more.

This is a memoir of a kid who came to the big city with big dreams and even bigger problems, only to find out that humanity is much more compassionate than he ever could have imagined.

It's about a guy who thought he had lost everything when he started to lose the color in his skin. This is one black man's story that is all about skin color, yet has absolutely nothing to do with racism.

It's about the disease that I thought would bring only misery and solitude. I say now, and I hope the pages of this book prove my point, that this ailment has brought me just the opposite.

Vitiligo has made me into the man I always wanted to be—and even more. This book tells the story of my journey— back to me. I don't know if that ever would have happened if I had not started turning white.

TWO

My Dream ... Deferred

LET'S TALK ABOUT DREAMS. They are the stuff that can make your heart pound. Just the thought of a dream becoming a reality can make you want to dance down the street or sing for no reason.

A dream is something vital to life—something that fuels our hopes.

I grew up with television, so maybe that's where my dreams came from. The same values as *Tarzan* and *The Rifleman* are mine. And I wanted to be smart like the Professor but have fun like Gilligan.

My dream was simple. I just wanted to be on TV. It seemed like that little box was my personal window on the world. It made everything exciting and fun while showing me anything was possible, even the wildest dreams like ...

Winning the lottery ...

Being in a movie ...

Even working on TV.

But what would happen if your dream came true?

I grew up the youngest of six kids in a military family. My father, a chief warrant officer, worked his way up the military ranks in the '60s and '70s.

At that time in America, what my father accomplished was no easy task. There was classism and racism and lots of pressures that always seemed to find their way back home. I believe it drove him to drink ... and to rule the house with the same iron fist he used on the job.

Mom was a housewife during my elementary school education. Then she became a nurse's aide after my parents divorced and we were struggling to make ends meet.

A lot of love and a lot of pain coexisted in the house as I was growing up. My parents both hail from the South. They dropped out of college because my dad enlisted and my mom followed him into a life in the military. And that was the beginning of the dreams deferred in the Thomas household. I'm referring to the Langston Hughes poem, *Dream Deferred*, in which he asks, "What happens to a dream deferred? Does it dry up like a raisin in the sun?" Maybe my parents' dreams were raisins, but I was determined to be different. Early on, I decided that I would follow my dreams to the bitter end.

It's funny, the things that stick in your head, but I remember the day. I was in junior high—seventh or eighth grade—and I wore these thick glasses. I was standing in the bathroom, which was the only private place most of the time in the house. And I took my glasses off, looked in the mirror, and decided right then and there that I was a handsome young man. And if that was true, why shouldn't all of my dreams come true?

So it was simple, I just needed to find a way to get rid of the glasses—then I was sure all of my hopes and wishes would become reality. I was already on the red carpet of my dreams, accepting the award for "Greatest TV Guy" when my brother interrupted my reverie:

"Where are my nunchucks?"

I had taken his karate fighting sticks! I had to leave the bathroom of dreams and make a run for it. I took off down the stairs, out the door. I kept running down the street before he figured out that I had them.

But before my mad dash, my decision was made. I would chase my dream no matter what—even if I was running from a sibling shortly after I made that life-defining choice.

Big Dreams in the Big Apple

I arrived at LaGuardia Airport after my first ride on an airplane as an adult. This was the big interview for the big job. I had just graduated from George Mason University in Fairfax, Virginia, just outside of Washington, D.C.

I worked at the TV station at school and eventually was promoted to produce and host my own show. That had prepared me to score this job interview for the kind of employment that I always expected. If I landed this job, I would be on a TV show in New York City.

From the time I boarded the plane at National Airport until the time I would return to Virginia, I wasn't going to miss a single second of what I hoped would be many New York "experiences." I had my camera and I was flashing pictures, one after another: the "Welcome to LaGuardia" sign outside the plane window as we glided in for touchdown; the interesting men in black, standing near baggage claim and holding signs with names on them. I remember thinking they must work for the government or they wouldn't be so dark and serious.

The company I was interviewing with said a car would be there to pick me up, but I didn't really know what that meant. I thought all those guys were butlers for the rich and famous— or G-men. So, I scanned the faces of the men in black waiting on superstars to see which one I would photograph first.

At the same time, I was looking for the lady I spoke with on the phone—the producer casting the show. I figured she would pick me up driving a Subaru or Toyota. As I scanned the faces, I had no idea what I might find.

Then, boom! There it was. There was a guy dressed in black with a white board that said, "Lee Thomas."

"Hey, man that's me," I yelled, like I just hit the Lotto or the man just called my winning bingo number. I was excited and with camera.

You know what that means—I took a picture of the guy. I took a picture of the sign. Then I had someone take a picture of the guy and the sign with me and my luggage. I did the same thing when we got to the nice Lincoln Town Car that was to take me into the city to my first job interview in NYC.

WWWOOOO!!!

I was on cloud nine ... with a camera. This was the first time in my life I actually had a driver who wasn't a parent, sibling, or classmate. I was far from my brother calling shotgun, leaving me to sit in the back of my mother's station wagon.

This was a real driver, man! I decided to sit in the back because that's what you do with a driver ... I thought.

By the way, when I got to the bottom of the escalator at the airport, I gave the guy a hug before I took pictures. I wasn't going to miss a moment of this stuff. Funny, I don't remember developing those shots, because I got the job and my life kicked into high gear.

World, I had just arrived! The year was 1991. I had made my dreams come true: a college degree and a job in New York City. Bliss, right? Well, it was for me. I got out of college and my first job in my chosen profession, television broadcasting, was in New York, the biggest media market in the United States of America. That's right, against all odds and shaking off the "real world" advice of my all professors, my friends, and basically everyone I met who had anything to do with TV. They all said there was no way I would ever get a job in New York right out of college. They were so wrong. And I was happy to be the one to prove them wrong.

I got the job. I think I wowed the show's executive producer with pure excitement. Now, I was in the Big Apple on a show called *Channel One.*

I was thinking, "OK, that's it. I'm going to be a big star."

But I didn't know how to write for TV. I didn't know how to read a teleprompter (I ad-libbed my college show). And I wasn't really sure what they wanted me to do. But I knew how to listen, learn, and turn it on for the camera. And I also knew how to turn it on for an interview. Because I love people.

It all happened so fast. Three weeks later, I was sharing an office in New York City. And I didn't know it then, but from the moment I walked through the door, my days on this show were numbered.

Channel One is a morning news program for middle and high school students. The show airs right in school just before first period. When I was there, the audience was eight million kids. *Channel One* was—and still is—the largest, guaranteed teen audience of any show in the United States.

The show was based in studios in New York City at 42nd Street and Third Avenue. It was a stone's throw from Grand Central Station. I could look out the office window and see a homeless guy begging in front of the building across the street. This was the concrete jungle I had heard about in so many rap songs and seen on countless TV shows. I wanted to know all about it.

But most of all, I just wanted to be successful.

About four months into my one-year contract, Jerry Liddel—who was the executive producer, a former executive with ABC's *Good Morning America*, and the man who hired me—called me into his office. He had promised to mentor me and help me grow. He had also told me not to worry about the bumps along the way. So, when he called me into the office, I really wasn't too concerned. I spoke to Jerry all the time, but once I got in and sat down, I knew this time would be different. He looked me straight in the eyes and said: "I

25

just want to tell you that I don't know if there's much more I can do for you."

"I'm fired," I said, with a lot of shock and the hint of a tear in my voice.

"No," he said, "I'm just saying I want you to do your best and don't let anyone here stop you."

"I will," I promised. "Jerry, is there something wrong?"

"No. How are things going, anyway?" His question steered the conversation into our usual topics. We would discuss my performance, the different producers, or the tough travel schedule. After that short scare, everything with the conversation seemed cool. ...

Until I came into work the next day. Jerry's office was clear. And I was in shock. Looking back, I understand what Jerry was doing. And I respect him for it—more than he probably knows. But at the time, I was a twenty-three-year-old broadcaster who was hungry to learn and expecting that my mentor would be there to help me along the journey. But yes, the next day, Jerry Liddel had been let go. His office was clear. He was gone.

It happened that quickly. And it was my first lesson in something that I know very well now: That's how TV works. One minute you're hot, the next minute you're fired. No hard feelings, it's the business.

A few weeks later, a new executive producer came in from Hollywood. He had what they called an MTV style. It was the new, hip way to do television. I was very interested in the new vision. I was excited to work with him and grow. But it seemed like as soon as he got there, I was sent on every out-of-town story that came along. Then, every time I was in town and tried to get a "sit-down, how am I doing?" meeting, his schedule was always too busy. Looking back after a decade or so in the business, I should have known something was up. But as a twenty-something young man living the dream, I didn't suspect anything. I figured if I worked hard, I would have no problems.

Once again, I needed someone to turn on the bright light of reality. And once again, someone I will never forget gave me a quick lesson in the ways of TV broadcasting. It was a reality check.

A couple of months into the new guy, one of the writer/ producers asked me to lunch. The producers never asked me to lunch, so I thought I must have done something right. The conversation that surrounded that meal changed my world.

We sat down and ordered.

"Do you have your resumé tape together?"

Once again, I was gripped with fear.

"What? Why?" All I needed to add was when, where,

how, and who, and I was the greatest reporter in the world. Could I have said anything any more inept?

"I know you're new to this," he said, "but you're a good guy, so I'm gonna break it down straight."

Next came one of those pauses ... you know, the kind where you know something that really sucks is about to follow.

"They're not going to renew your contract."

I was floored.

"When the guy who hires you gets fired," he explained in a matter-of-fact TV News 101 voice, "the new guy comes in to revamp the show. Besides getting a new set or a new look for the broadcast, the first thing to change is the faces—the anchors and the reporters. You are one of the faces."

I was silent.

"Don't take it personally," he said. "Spend a few days getting your resumé tape together. Because when the new guy drops the hammer, it may be quick, and you may not be let back into the building. And by the way, it may be before the end of the month."

Wow, just like that, my dream was gone. Lucky for me, the end didn't come as quickly as it could have. Over the next month, I tried to meet with the new guy, but he was still too busy. And they kept sending me out of town. When I finally did corner him, he reassured me without ever mentioning my contract being renewed. I almost believed I had a chance. He was smooth. I call it "the Los Angeles way." It's a way of saying something bad in a fashion that sounds good. Just before summer, I got the news. My time there was done. The show hit the summer hiatus and I still had two months left on my contract. I was told I was not getting renewed, but I would still receive full pay through the term of the deal. That made me happy; I had more time to regroup. Plus, I would get some time to digest what had just happened.

Did I blow my big dream? And what would I do next? Little did I know that at the time, the emotional and physical toll from that loss would be immeasurable.

But I swore to keep fighting. And I did.

Muhammad and Me

"Float like a butterfly, stink on TV, no one is as bad a reporter as me." I love to rhyme.

It was a brisk day as the wind slid off the Ohio River. And even though I was there shooting a story on the man the world simply calls "The Greatest," I came up with the poem. Why? Because I couldn't help but think how a young Cassius Clay must have felt after he watched his dream sink to the bottom of the river.

I was standing on Second Street Bridge in Louisville, Kentucky. History had documented that as the place where the man who would become Muhammad Ali threw his Olympic gold medal into the depths of the swirling water below. The story goes, after coming home from winning the Olympic light heavyweight boxing title, Ali could not get served at a diner in his hometown of Louisville because of the color of his skin. As a result, the insulted champion came to the bridge and threw the medal in the river. It was a dream that the man had literally fought for and won. Now, the embodiment of that dream—the gold medal—was gone, and Ali was changed forever. It did not stop him. He would rise to even greater heights than any athlete in the history of this country.

But the disappointment in that moment, that's dramatic stuff. And that's how I felt leaving New York. My dream had sunk to the bottom of my heart. And I had to find a way to tread water until I could stage a comeback.

I lost the dream job before I even really knew what I was doing. But because of the advice from some very nice people, I was ready. I made a resumé tape before I was no longer allowed in the building. I had also decided it was time for me to go in a specific direction—entertainment reporting. I had gotten a taste of it by doing some feature stories at *Channel One*. So I sent a tape to the only entertainment show I could find in the country with a job opening. It was in Louisville, Kentucky. *Louisville Tonight Live* was the local version of *Entertainment Tonight* and one of the last *PM Magazine*-style local entertainment and feature shows in the United States.

I got the job! After a whirlwind first year in the business in New York, Louisville offered my first opportunity to rest and catch up with my emotions. And it wasn't easy. I didn't know anyone. I would go out with co-workers, talk to the girls, play basketball, or just lay in my bed and stare at the ceiling. I believed I could figure out the "why?" of what happened in New York.

My heart was aching for the dream I felt had been snatched away for reasons I did not understand.

I tried to get up off the bed, and suddenly I felt hurt in another way: Knife-like pain zigzagged through my lower back.

I lay back down until it went away. I just figured it was not time to get up ... even though staring at the ceiling was a great practice in meditation.

Finally, after a few months, I was able to stop thinking about what happened in New York. I didn't understand it any better, I just put it away so I could do my new job. And even though I was far from the "Muhammad Ali" of reporters, I decided I would try to be "the greatest" entertainment reporter who ever lived. Or I would just do my best to keep my job and move up in the industry as quickly as I could. Thankfully, the job was everything I wanted it to be. I interviewed celebrities who came to town. I got to do stories on movies and events. But most of all, this show was all about live television. While *Channel One* was taped, this was the real deal—live TV with in-field reporting and on-set interaction with the hosts. This was my first taste of spontaneous talk. And I knew right away that this was my thing.

Louisville became home. And it didn't take very long. It's funny, I learned a lot from my experience there. And I would always use "the champ" as inspiration. I would fight my way back into broadcasting one punch at a time. Eventually I would "shake up the world."

Ali was straight inspiration, even though I recently learned that the whole gold-medal-in-the-water story was not true. The current version of history is that he just lost it. Not as glamorous nor as big a statement against the state of American life. But no matter how it went down, the result for me was the same. I was inspired to work hard for my dream. No matter how many punches it took, literally and figuratively, Ali always fought back and won. I would adopt that philosophy. But it was in Louisville that I got the first counterpunch in the toughest fight in my life. Just down the street and around the corner from the Second Street Bridge, in a neighborhood barbershop, my new fight began.

The First Sight of White

I used to go with what's called "the DC fade." It was a college-boy haircut that was very popular in Washington, D.C. That clean-cut look had served me so well in college. But now I was trying to be different. I was trying to be a grown-up. So, I went to the barbershop to get the proper haircut—one that was appropriate for a young reporter. I decided to go with "the skin fade"—no hair on the side and very short hair on top. You can still see scalp all over, but the haircut is very clean. This haircut is a favorite among soldiers. When the barber finished, he pulled off the tape and put the stinking alcohol around the edge. I was in the chair, talking with the fellas, when the barber handed me a hand mirror. Something was wrong.

It looked like he had taken out a chunk of my hair. "What's that, man?" I asked with a tone that implied he had messed up. "You nicked me!"

"No, I didn't," he said.

I was fully expecting not to pay him for this bad hair job. "Then what's that?" I accused.

"It's a white spot on your scalp," he said. I did an in-depth investigation. The man was right. A white spot—about one inch by one and a half inches—marked my scalp on the back of my head. A few smaller, less noticeable specks of white surrounded the big spot.

"It's a stress mark," the barber said. "It'll probably just go away."

I had gone through a lot in the last few months—changing jobs, changing cities, and going from the number one city in the world to the forty-sixth biggest city in the nation. I figured I was lucky to have only one little stress-related mark. So I didn't think much of it.

All of twenty-four years old, I thought, "This, too, shall pass." That's something my mom used to say. I felt even more reassured after speaking with one of my friends from college. He said the same thing happened to him. A white spot appeared on his scalp, and then disappeared a few months later.

Right then, I stopped thinking about it. And I did what I always do. I focused my attention on my work. The new job was fun and a great place to learn TV. I was happy, but still eager to get back and take my bite out of the Big Apple.

Amazingly, the chance came much sooner and in a bigger way than I had hoped.

And this time, I was ready.

New York Again

Louisville was an excellent training ground for my triumphant return to New York. I viewed the Midwestern city as a big small town where I was happy to work and learn. Thankfully, I did so under the guidance of folks like George Hultcher, the station manager who hired me. A TV veteran who came from big markets like Philly and New York, he ruled the station like it was a vacation for him. Wearing deck shoes and polo shirts most days, his relaxed approach to television was a welcoming comfort and just what I needed. He taught me how to write and perform.

But most of all, he taught me that TV wasn't about me. It was about the people and their stories. I was the conduit making the information accessible—and sometimes entertaining. That's the biggest lesson I received from my man, George. I was doing well and learning every day. So I just kept doing my job, trying to get better. And I was always thinking that one day, if I were lucky, I could go back and reclaim New York as my broadcasting turf—never to be exiled again.

I also hired myself a big-time agent. She would focus on the next job while I concentrated on working harder and longer. "When I get back, I will be unstoppable," I told myself. That's really what I thought; I was only twenty-four years old.

Then about eight or nine months into my job, the call came. My agent said it was a big station in New York. They were looking for a new entertainment reporter, and the news director was interested in me.

Yes! I wanted it bad. And from the moment my agent brought it up, the only place I could find answers was from my good friend, the ceiling in my room. I couldn't tell my co-workers everything. This is a competitive business.

But the ceiling would tell no lies, pull no punches, and keep its mouth shut ... since, you know, it didn't have a mouth. So, I played "what if" in my head. I just knew if it came through, I would work so hard, I would die before I let this job slip away.

Months went by and I heard nothing about the job. I passed the one-year mark in Kentucky and still no word about the job in New York. I would go to the library and look through *Broadcasting Magazine*, the industry bible, every week, just to see what was out there. And one day I saw a listing from the same station. They were looking for a general assignment reporter. I wanted to do entertainment, but the listing was for straight news. I sent my tape anyway, just to remind them that I was available. A week later, I was sitting at my desk writing a story when the phone rang.

"*Louisville Tonight*, this is Lee, may I help you?"

"Is this Lee Thomas?"

"Yes."

"This is Henry Florsheim, news director of WABC in New York. How are you?"

I was back!

Two weeks later, I was sitting in his office. He offered me the job on the elevator as we rode down to get the car and return to the airport for my flight back to Louisville. Two months later, I was sitting at my desk in the WABC newsroom and the wrong was now right.

I was living my dream at my new work home, the ABC building on 67th Street on the west side of Manhattan. It was the greatest job in the world! The station shared a studio with *Live with Regis and Kathy Lee*, a real syndicated morning show. Now *that* was the job I really wanted: hosting a show. I decided to watch Regis' every move (and Gelman's, the show's producer). I poured myself into the job. I spent twelve hours a day and even weekends laboring at this dream job.

As for food, the faster the better. I had no time to prepare meals. Being young and healthy, I saw no reason to even *think* about my diet. My only concern was that it was quick, tasty, and filling. My nutritional nightmare kicked off every morning with I called "the big nasty." The first time I ate one, I said, "This is the best cinnamon roll I've ever had in my life! I've gotta eat one every day!"

And I practically did, with a large cup of tea. I'd buy the big nasty from one of those carts on Manhattan street corners that sell steaming-hot coffee and melt-in-your-mouth, monster-sized bagels. But the bagels weren't as big as my cinnamon rolls. These gooey concoctions of dough, frosting, and spice were enormous—like a small Frisbee. With that giant sugar/flour glob in my gut, I would dash to the TV studios to get my assignments for the day. Then I'd be all over the media capital of world, reporting on the hottest entertainment stories.

Lunchtime meant a stop at a local bodega, one of the small shops in the city's ethnic neighborhoods. They offered these incredible buffets with everything you can imagine. I mostly dived into Chinese chicken dishes, washed down with plenty of Mountain Dew or Dr Pepper. Another lunchtime favorite was the meatball submarine sandwich at Subway.

The healthiest meals I ate were usually in the ABC cafeteria in our building. It was subsidized, so I could get a full meal—like baked turkey, dressing, vegetables, salad, a drink, and a piece of cake—all for about four bucks!

Dinner took me to this authentic Mexican restaurant near my apartment for the most enormous burritos you've ever seen. The size of a head of lettuce, they were stuffed with meat, cheese, and all the fixin's that make burritos so delicious. I was a big chicken guy, so I'd also get their chicken con carne with ham and sauce. Fried chicken from other restaurants was a favorite, too.

Wait, my Texas-sized consumption in the Big Apple didn't end with dinner.

"Hey, aren't you that guy from TV?" strangers would say if I walked into a bar, club, or restaurant in the evening. "Let me buy you a drink!"

Or two or three. Rum and Coke, vodka and cranberry juice, or vodka and citron flowed freely down my throat on many evenings.

All this yummy food and drink on the go kept my taste buds happy. I made no connection between my high-fat, high-sugar, low-fiber diet and that recurring pain in my back. I was too busy working to think about the pain ... the white spots on my scalp ... or my state of extreme fatigue. Plus, I had a girlfriend, whom I met through a mutual friend. So any time that I wasn't working or sleeping, I was romancing my girl, who had a cool New York job in design.

I had it all on a silver platter in the greatest city on Earth.

And I would not fail! I would die of overwork before I would let that happen ... again.

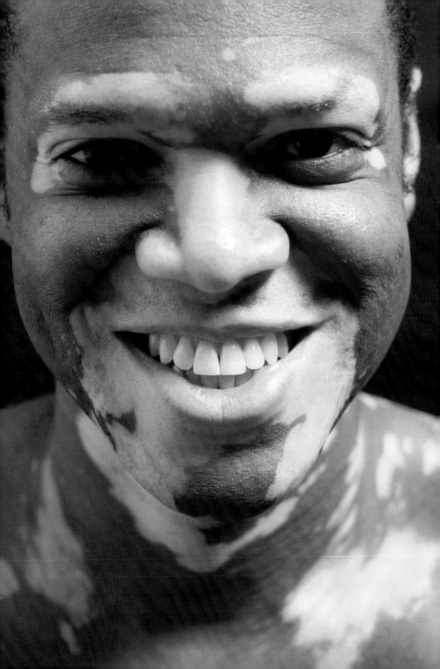

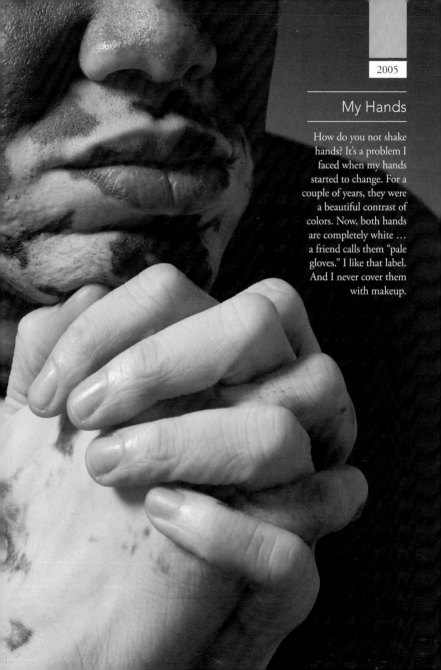

2005

My Hands

How do you not shake hands? It's a problem I faced when my hands started to change. For a couple of years, they were a beautiful contrast of colors. Now, both hands are completely white … a friend calls them "pale gloves." I like that label. And I never cover them with makeup.

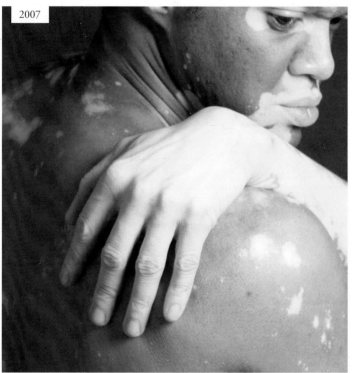

2007

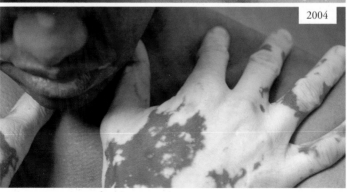

2004

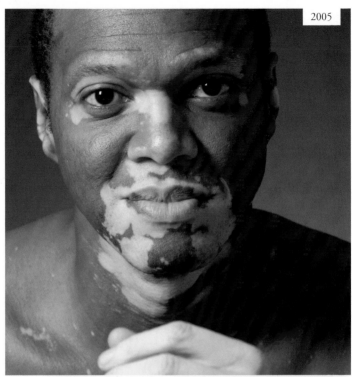
2005
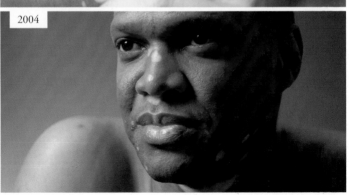
2004

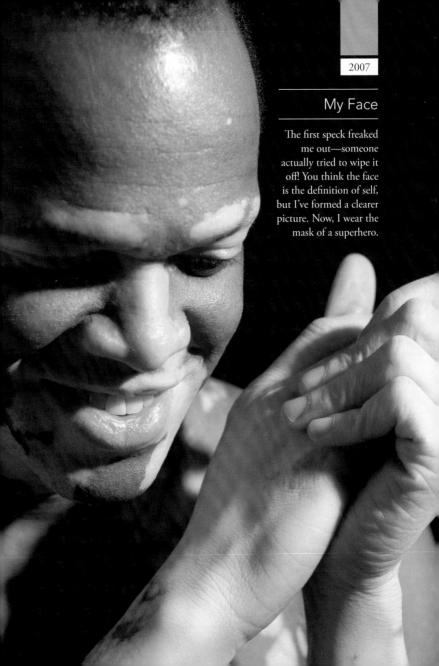

My Face

The first speck freaked me out—someone actually tried to wipe it off! You think the face is the definition of self, but I've formed a clearer picture. Now, I wear the mask of a superhero.

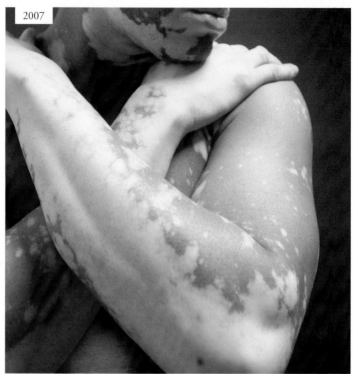

2007

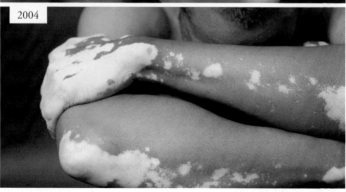

2004

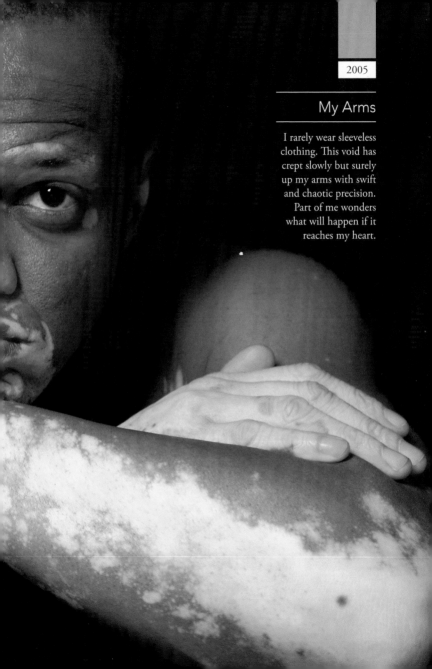

2005

My Arms

I rarely wear sleeveless clothing. This void has crept slowly but surely up my arms with swift and chaotic precision. Part of me wonders what will happen if it reaches my heart.

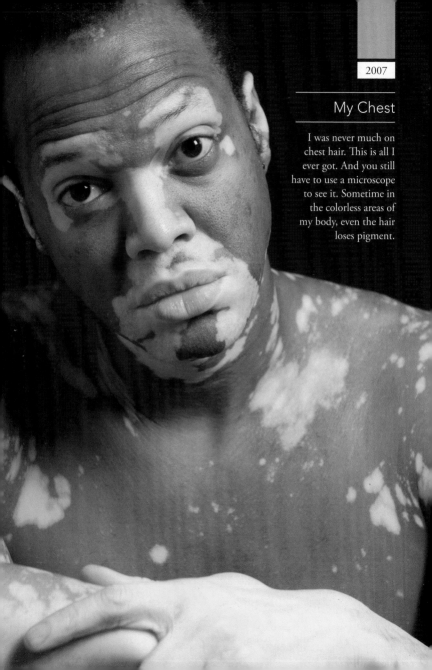

2007

My Chest

I was never much on chest hair. This is all I ever got. And you still have to use a microscope to see it. Sometime in the colorless areas of my body, even the hair loses pigment.

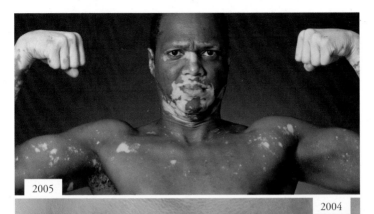

2005

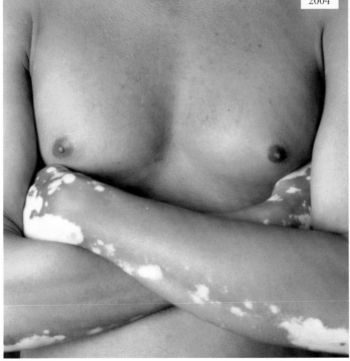

2004

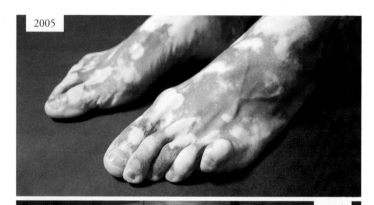

2005

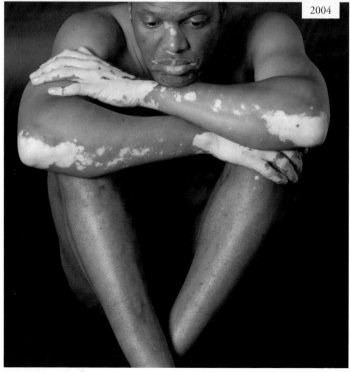

2004

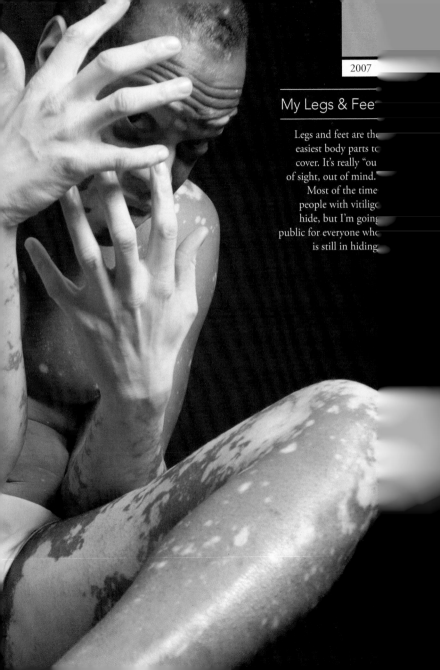

2007

My Legs & Fee[t]

Legs and feet are the
easiest body parts to
cover. It's really "ou[t]
of sight, out of mind."
Most of the time
people with vitilig[o]
hide, but I'm going
public for everyone wh[o]
is still in hiding.

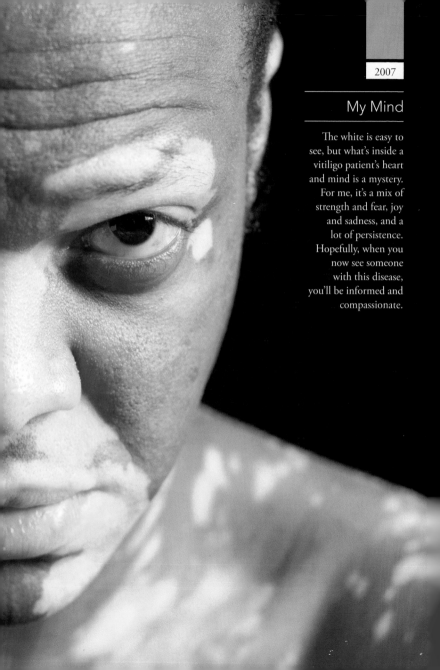

2007

My Mind

The white is easy to
see, but what's inside a
vitiligo patient's heart
and mind is a mystery.
For me, it's a mix of
strength and fear, joy
and sadness, and a
lot of persistence.
Hopefully, when you
now see someone
with this disease,
you'll be informed and
compassionate.

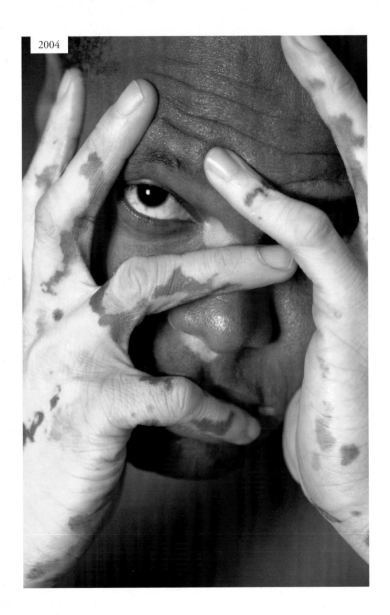

2004

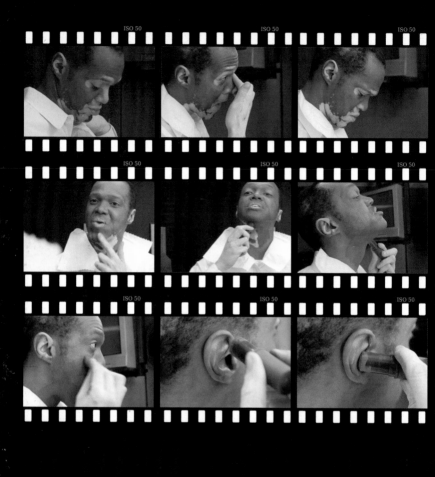

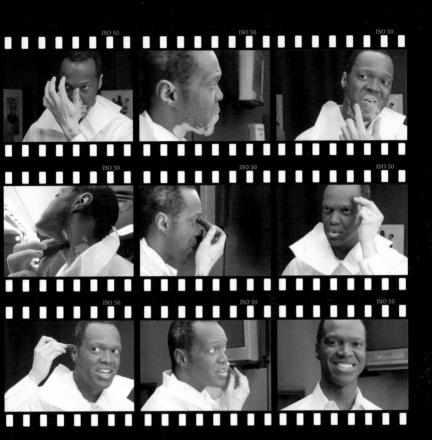

Makeup in the Morning

This is where the magic happens. It takes about twenty minutes to put on my makeup every morning. I even have to put it on my ears. A newscast is about the information. My face would make every story about me, so I cover up. It's a small price to pay to do the job I love.

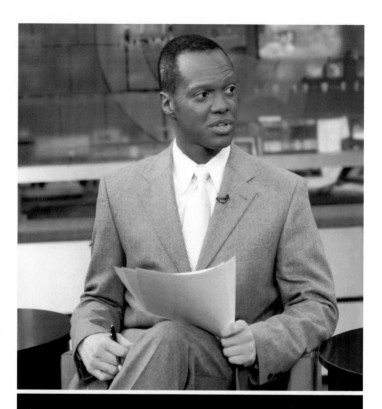

On the Set

I worked hard to be in this chair. It took me a long time to understand that being a broadcaster is about other people. We share in heartache and drama, love and happiness. We put words to moments that can be life changing. We record and chronicle history. Thanks for sharing in mine.

PHOTOGRAPHS BY MICHAEL SHORE

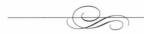

THREE

Searching for Home

"LOOK AT THAT BIG OLD HOG HEAD!"

I wasn't talking about Arnold the pig from the '60s TV show, *Green Acres*. I was looking at a tape of one of my reports. I was sure the collar of that shirt was just screaming at my neck to give it a break. It was straining its top button, barely holding all that neck in place without popping.

I had gained weight, but I was too tired to weigh myself.

This happened about a year into the job after I had a stretch of nonstop work that was about five weeks long. I mean five weeks straight, including weekends. I had not taken a day off for five weeks, and I didn't even notice until the third week! I did notice something was also a little peculiar.

I was always tired. From the moment I woke up until the moment I returned home, I was exhausted.

In the midst of fatigue and weight gain, I decided to look at that white area on my scalp. The last time I had looked, the spot had gotten smaller. Now I just wanted to make sure it was still going away. But much to my surprise—or should I call it shock and horror?—the white spot on my scalp had multiplied to three spots! And white specks were forming on my hand.

That's when I found a dermatologist. The man who diagnosed the vitiligo and informed me, "There is no cure."

That night, when I returned to my small studio apartment that I could barely afford, the ceiling welcomed me like an old friend. It was pure white and I almost felt like I was staring into my future.

That gave me a weird sense of comfort because it was the only place where I felt I would be able to share my problems. I could release all of my newfound challenges to the white abyss. There were no obligations or ramifications. The ceiling was a silent and trustworthy confidant.

We shared many things to analyze beyond the surface.

Yes, I have an incurable disease. But it was even deeper than the white spots. Why this disease? Why so visual, so personal to my career? There has to be some kind of message.

It's not fatal, so this is something I have been chosen to live with. I could have gotten any disease, but I have this? Maybe it symbolizes something that I need to acknowledge. It is presenting lessons I need to learn. It is now part of my life's journey to recognize these lessons, address them, and grow. Or will the lessons keep coming until I grow?

What does it mean to turn white with a disease that comes with no explanation for why it happens? And no remedy for a cure? Well, the doctor did say it could be triggered by stress. And the way I was working was very, very stressful. The heart-pounding, adrenaline rush and anxiety of deadlines constantly loomed. Add to that the critical eyes of millions of people watching my every move and listening to my every word.

Even more stressful was the fact that I was in a building right next to the network offices, where every executive had a television on his desk. Which meant that from the president of ABC all the way down the chain of command to my boss, they were all watching every broadcast, every day, without question. And if by chance something were to go wrong, as soon as you got back to your desk in the newsroom, someone would call you into their office before you could sit down. Or as soon as you sat down and began to work, your phone would ring.

And it could be any of them.

One day I got off the air thinking I did a decent job.

My phone rang. The lady at the other end said, "This is the office of Roone Arledge calling for Lee Thomas."

I instantly soiled my shorts, figuratively. Roone Arledge was the head of the network, the man who came up with the concept for *The Wide World of Sports*. He's the guy who hired broadcasting legend Howard Cosell and created *Monday Night Football*. Arledge could make or break your career.

So after I checked my shorts, I said, "This is Lee." This call could be really bad or really good; there was no in between.

And then the woman asked, "Is this the Lee Thomas who's a network cameraman?"

I answered in a tone of both relief and disappointment: "No, I'm the reporter with *Eyewitness News*."

"Sorry for the inconvenience," she said.

As I caught my breath, I realized how tightly wound I had become. I had already messed up a couple of times and gotten into an argument with the assignment editor. I also came through big a couple of times, but the workload and the stress were taking their toll.

Man, I felt like I was about to break. I was chronically tired. I didn't even know what watching my diet meant. My girlfriend got a great job in Los Angeles, so she moved to the opposite side of the country. And of course, now I had these white spots. It was time to do something, but first I had to go to the bathroom before I left a wet spot in my chair.

When I got home that night, the ceiling and I had a heart-to-heart. I really needed to do something or I wasn't only going to turn white, I felt like I was about to fade out completely. I had chronic fatigue. I mean, I was just plain old tired and it would not go away—even after I had a weekend off. I was so busy trying to be what *they* wanted me to be and hold on to my opportunity, that I wasn't sure if I was being what *I* wanted to be.

The opportunity was huge and the job was daunting. I had worked five weeks straight and all I had to show for it was the fact that I had gained fifteen pounds. I know that because I had finally gotten to the gym and weighed myself. I was the heaviest I had ever been in my life. And I was starting to look bad. The tape of one of my reports was not lying. My head and neck were bigger, and I looked tired, with baggy eyes, hog head, and all. My collar was so tight, it looked like my neck was spilling out of my shirt, and the tie was just hanging there, trying to get away. So when I got on the scale at the gym ...

Wow! How could I have gained that much weight and not even notice?

What to do, what to do. I can't quit! This is the chance of a lifetime. I will try to eat better and work out more.

So, I did try. But it was tough.

Here's a sample of a daily schedule: I would wake up around 6:30 a.m. to prepare for the day, then walk to work to arrive by 8 a.m. I would get my story for the day, then go and shoot it with one of the cameramen. Sometimes I would shoot two stories in a day. And even though Manhattan is a small island, all of New York City's viewing audience is everywhere—from Long Island to Jersey. Getting a story done was no easy task. Drive time alone could be the biggest challenge.

After I would shoot a story, I had to get back and write. Then send it to an editor. And make sure it's produced well and ready to present on that evening's newscast. I would usually come back, write, and get into editing by 3:30 or 4 p.m. All the while, I would be making phone calls throughout the day to find future stories and make contacts that would give me great stuff later.

Editing required at least an hour and a half. Then it was time to prepare to go on the air live in the 5 p.m. newscast. I would be finished by 6 p.m. Then it was time to prep for the next day. Since it was my job to stay up on entertainment, I would then go to a show or a movie that would start by 7 or 8 p.m. and be over around 9 or 10 p.m. I attended shows at least three nights a week and once on weekends.

At the same time, I was always scanning information to

make sure I had not missed any stories. Nothing could exist on the entertainment landscape of the city I didn't know about. I was on the same newscast as a well-respected movie reviewer named Joel Siegel and a well-connected lifestyles reporter named Judy Licht. I was just trying to keep up with the people in my office, not to mention the rest of the city. Think of it as treading water, trying to keep from drowning in a busy pool of entertainment broadcasting.

My job was my life. I would, however, try to find time to play basketball during my scarce free time. Man, it was a grind. There was no time to really eat. Many of my meals were grab and go. Despite all of the pressures and problems, I always reminded myself that this was my dream job. I'd lost it once before and was lucky enough to get a second chance, all before age twenty-five! I was defying the odds in every way, so I could deal with the drawbacks.

I would never give up!

But the ceiling was telling me something very different. All that white space had a way of firing off so many relevant questions.

"What if you turn white?"

"Can you cover it with makeup?"

"And if you can cover it up, is that something you even want to do?"

"What if your boss sees you turning white and fires you?"
Damn you, ceiling! Shut up!

Getting a Grip

Television is a vapid visual medium, which meant that if I didn't lose weight, deal with my white spots, and cure my chronic fatigue, my dream would end before it had really gotten started. Because I intended to do TV for a long, long time, it was time for Lee Thomas to work hard at getting healthy. And I knew just where to start.

I started my change by going on a ten-day fast called "the master cleanser." It was a lemon juice diet that all of the models in NYC were trying. And a friend gave me the book. She said it helped her with fatigue. I lost fourteen pounds. But it was very tough to skip lunch. I use to share a lunch with a longtime news writer/producer who would tell me stories of old. I loved our lunches, but I couldn't eat with him for a while during this fast. And I couldn't go in the network cafeteria. It would just be too tempting.

Instead my meals consisted of lemon juice mixed with maple syrup and cayenne pepper. It was hard; at times I felt really weak. But after the ten days were over, I felt great. And for about a week, my energy came back. Even the spot on my hand was showing signs of pigment. I was excited.

So I plugged myself back into my job. I even enjoyed brief moments of happiness. But a month later, I found myself skipping movies and going home to bed. I was tired again. And the white spots started to grow. I returned to the dermatologist; he gave me some cream that was different from the last cream. That's when I went back to my trusted friend, the ceiling. It was a different ceiling because I had moved from a high-rise studio (with an alcove) to a one bedroom in Park Slope, Brooklyn.

In my old place on the west side of Manhattan, it had cost me an extra two hundred dollars per month to have a six foot by eight foot alcove just off the bathroom. It's New York.

But the change was comforting because the ceiling in Brooklyn must have known the ceiling in Manhattan, or maybe they knew some of the same fixtures, because they both seemed to be saying the same thing:

"You have a great job that's not making you happy."

"You look like you're in great shape, but you're turning white and you're always tired."

"And what about those scary back pains?"

"Maybe the problem and the answer are the same."

"It's you."

Well, at first I thought the ceiling was crazy. Then it began to sink in. I was the only one pushing myself to work this hard. No one in the office was telling me I had to know and do everything. It was me. When it finally sunk in, it was a shock. I couldn't believe the ceiling was right. Was it telling me to leave my great job?

"Are you happy?"

I'll be damned. The answer was: "No."

And a year and a half into one of the best opportunities in my life, I decided that I had to leave.

"Are you sure?"

I heard that from many of my friends when I told them my intentions. I know they thought I was crazy leaving the job of a lifetime. But I was on a journey, not just to find another job. That would not be good enough. I needed to find my happiness. My head and neck may have been back to normal size, but I still was not healthy. I could feel it. Therefore, I needed to find my health. I would start the journey with a simple mission. Health and happiness! No matter what anyone said, I would try to start all over.

Only in L.A. Story

I got to the gym and wrote my name on the sign-up board.

"Next!" called the street ballers, who announce that word like no others.

At the Hollywood YMCA back in 1997, you signed your

name and you played with the other four names on the board that were next.

Playing here on the West Coast was a little different than the courts in New York, or even back in Louisville. Further east, you call, "Next!" and pick your team. But I was a visitor here, so home team ruled. I just wanted to play some ball and have fun.

I had left New York for a multitude of reasons. I thought the main one was to be with my girlfriend, who had moved to L.A. to work on a sitcom. I wanted to see if it would work with her. My girl was a very talented costume designer, and she was working hard to make it in show business.

I was also trying to figure out a direction for my career and navigate the whole health thing. I wanted to fuel up and not be tired anymore. I wanted to love her and find my health. I had just left a great job by choice, and now I wanted something in my life to work. So I thought I would start with love and maybe the job and the health thing would come around.

I was sitting courtside, watching the game. I looked at the board and saw the names of the guys who would be on my team. I heard names being called back and forth on and off the court. I was trying to size up the guys. I wanted to see if the people I was playing with were any good.

Then I saw a name high on the board: "Denzel." He must have played already. It couldn't be the actor, though. This was Hollywood, but it was the YMCA in Hollywood. And I was looking at the court and didn't recognize any A-List stars. One of the guys on the winning team must have had the same name. I wondered if he was black. "I've never met a white Denzel," I thought, as I went in the other room to stretch.

Whose momma named a guy Denzel? And it must suck to be in Hollywood with that name and not be a star. "Hi, I'm Denzel Herzog." Yep, that would suck for him—but I needed to stretch because I didn't want to just run one game and sit.

Street ball rules are pretty much the same everywhere you play. It's simple. Play, you stay. Lose, you cruise. Translation: As long as you win, your team stays on the court to play all challengers. If you lose, your name goes back on the list and you have to wait your turn again.

Well, I had all day. I was "between projects" right now. That was a term I learned the day before. It's the Hollywood way of saying, "I have no job." I wanted to win so I could play without sitting.

"Yo, Lee!" a dude shouted. "Is Lee in here?"

"Yep," I answered.

"You're up, man! Better come with it 'cause these guys been on all day."

It was my turn to play. And I wanted to win. I walked into the gym and the dude said, "You got him, you straight?" (Translation: He was asking me if I could guard the man. I can guard anybody, so naturally I told him I was ready.)

I looked over at this scruffy guy with a short, messed-up Afro and a unkempt beard. He was about five-foot-eleven and kinda wide.

No problem, I think.

"No problem, ball up top," I said. Let's play.

Then the scruffy guy opened his mouth, "Ball up top."

And I heard a *Crimson Tide/Malcolm X* voice. I looked up. I'll be damned!

Behind all that unkempt beard was a man who owned an Oscar. Yes, I was guarding the real Denzel Washington. Maybe his scruffy look was for a movie or something.

"What's up?" I said, trying to play it cool.

"Hope you came to play." He tossed me the ball and said, "Ball in," and I gave it back, which meant we were ready to play. The action would start once he threw the ball to a teammate. And that's what he did. He quickly threw the ball in, then ran past me for a give-and-go. That means you pass the ball to a teammate and cut to the basket, then he passes it back and you score. His player threw the ball back to him and he had an easy layup. Denzel Washington can ball! And he just scored on me! I wasn't sure if I should laugh or be mad or call my mom. She would get a kick out of this one. But my star-struck daze didn't last very long.

On the way back up court, Mr. Washington smiled. As he got into position to guard me, he said, "Are you gonna guard me or watch?" Damn, not only can he ball, but he scored on me, and he talks trash! I love this man! I wanted to give him some dat right then and there. (Dat is the universal handshake that black men share among themselves and with others.) Until one of my teammate's words smacked me back into reality. "Can you handle him or what? Game is to twelve."

Oh, yeah, if we lost, I would have to sit back down and wait for another thirty or forty minutes to get back on the court. So, I had better play ball to win no matter who was the opponent. So, I manned up.

Denzel, Shmenzel. It was time to play ball. So I was playing the backside and I saw a clear cut to the lane. If my man passed me the ball, I would have Denzel beat for an easy basket. So, I went.

But as I went, I felt something holding onto my shirt. It was Denzel. He wouldn't let me go. I had him beat, but the man was holding my shirt. And he was smiling. The Oscar winner was not only holding my shirt and slowing me up so I couldn't cut the lane, he was also laughing about it. Ain't that a bitch? I knocked his hand off and cut. But it was too late. One of his guys stepped in a grabbed the pass. It was a turnover. At that point, he was laughing and I was ticked. So this was what L.A. was like. Was this some kind of weird welcome?

Well, I had a little welcome myself. I don't care if it's Denzel or the president of the country. This was basketball and we are both men. Therefore, I will not be clowned by anyone. Let the games begin.

Denzel got the ball on offense and did a quick move to try and get the easy layup on me again. This time I had to stage a *Siege* for mister *John Q*. Oh, yeah baby, it was *Training Day*. I'd make sure *He Got Game*. A lot of game. So I fouled him. I fouled him hard. That was mean. I swatted the ball and his arm, knocking him out of bounds. But not hard enough to hurt the man. Come on, it was Denzel. I tapped him hard enough to let him know that I was there and the easy shot stuff was over. He and the ball went out of bounds. Then I smiled at him. He smiled back and the game was on. His team ended up winning, but it was fun. It made me like him even more.

And I should have known that with that as my introduction to Los Angeles, it was going to be an interesting time with many surprises and lots of fun. The game was strangely symbolic of my entire time in Los Angeles. I would have fun and get knocked around a little bit. But I was never really sure if I was winning or losing.

The first of the surprises was that I really wasn't sleeping well and the L.A. ceiling looked funny. Plus, my girlfriend would grind her teeth at night as she slept. Then she refused to believe me when I told her it was happening. So I started to think that I was crazy. She had never done that in New York. I guess the stress of trying to make it in Hollywood was getting to her. Or maybe it was having me around again. She was a very smooth character while she was awake, but things happen in your sleep that you can't control.

Another thing I couldn't control was her stuff. Or should I say, her lack of stuff. When I got to her place, she had no TV, no couch—not even a bed.

I didn't have a car. I would take the bus to the gym because she needed her car, and that would be the extent of my day. So, after I got my bearings straight, I used some of the money I had saved and bought a little truck, a couch, a bed, and a TV. I thought she would be happy but she didn't really seem to care about the stuff.

I didn't understand that at the time, but I do now. She was so focused on her job that everything else didn't really matter. And I think our relationship was part of the stuff that didn't matter. I mean, don't get me wrong. She loved me and

I loved her, but she loved her career more. And I really needed to find some stable ground. It's not her fault, but the longer I stayed there, the only thing that got better was my basketball skills. I got pretty good while between jobs.

I also tried to eat better and find some healthy alternatives that I hoped would cure my white spot problem. By the way, at the time I only had a couple of spots on my scalp and a couple on one of my hands.

Detroit Keeps Calling

After I had been in the City of Angels for a little over a month, nothing was going on except basketball. So I let my new agent know that I was looking to get some work or at least some interviews. Management of my career had been taken over by the owner of the agency. He was well-known and as powerful as they come in the world of broadcast news. Within days, I got a call from my man about a job. A news director in Detroit wanted me to do sports.

I don't do sports. I do entertainment. So thanks, but no thanks.

The agent also set me up with an interview at a local Los Angeles station. It was weird. The newsroom was inside one of the stages on a studio lot. I didn't get a good feeling from the place, and they never offered me the job. After a few days, my agent called back. Now the guy in Detroit wanted me to do weather.

I'm not a meteorologist. Nor do I wish to fake being one on TV. So once again, thanks, but no thanks.

I knew what I wanted—a top ten city and a job where I could do live feature and entertainment stuff and learn how to be a great morning anchor.

Don't get me wrong. I was flattered with the offer. But if I've learned one thing about this business, it's don't take a job that's less than what you want. Wait, and what you really want will eventually come.

And it did. A week or so later, another call.

"What, Detroit again?"

"No, Showtime (network) wants you in New York to audition to host a free weekend."

"Hey!" I exclaimed, "now that sounds awesome. Except I'm in L.A. and I can't just fly to NYC for an audition with no guarantee of work. And they're not going to pay for the trip. I hate to keep saying this, but no thanks."

I was starting to think that all of the jobs that people were looking at me for were things just beyond my reach for one reason or another. Around about now, the big mental doubts started kicking in. I had been in La La Land nearly two months. My girl and I weren't doing badly, but we definitely were not doing well, either. I was just kinda there. Plus, I couldn't get any work.

Forget the ceiling. I would find myself during the day just staring at the wall, waiting for the time to go to the gym. I reserved the ceiling for the nighttime analysis. And since I had advanced to daytime mental abuse, the wall would do just fine. One afternoon I was staring at the wall so hard that my brow was wrinkled. It was so tight that I was getting a headache. Then the phone rang. It was my agent. Detroit was back. This time the man wanted me to be a weekend anchor and do feature reports during the week. Now this was something I could work with.

And the call got even better. "Oh, yeah," my agent said, "You don't need an audition. Showtime wants you for the job. You go to Vancouver in two weeks."

"Are they going to pay me?"

"That's why I'm here."

"Then I'll get my passport and I'll talk to you more about the Detroit thing later. Thanks."

Just like that, I was back. I just got an assignment and didn't even have to audition. Plus, a potential job offer. So the wall must have more power than the ceiling. There's a lot to be said for just sitting up.

Anyway, things were starting to look up. I would go

to Vancouver. My trip would give my girl a break from me sitting around staring at her walls. Plus, I could have some fun and think about my next move. I didn't know anything about Detroit, but I decided it couldn't hurt to take a trip up there and see.

Judge the Book and Cover

I woke up in another hotel room and took a look around to try and figure out where I was. They all look the same. I had just finished the four-day trip to Canada, so I couldn't be there anymore. And my girl wasn't by my side, so I wasn't in L.A.

As I stumbled to the bathroom, I saw my favorite suit in the closet. That's when reality hit. This was the land of Marvin Gaye; UAW country. I was in a place they call the Motor City and Motown, but to me it was just plain old Detroit.

I had no impression. I was here to analyze a potential job. I still had money and a girl who loved me back in Hollywood. This job would have to be good for me to change my life. I was indifferent to the change.

After I finished in the bathroom, I decided to tune into the newscast on which I might be working. I never should have done that. The anchors were OK, but the set look like it was straight out of 1977. They were also a very bland version of news—no frills, and no fun ... just news.

The show was all about business and cold hard reality. No joking, no flexibility, no off-the-cuff. Which meant no me. I had made my name as a fun and light-hearted feature and entertainment guy. I was best at spontaneous fun. That show appeared to have no place for a guy like me. It was one of those love or hate deals.

My presence would either be the burst of sunshine they needed, or it would be, "Where did that come from? And when is it going back?"

Still, I put on my power suit. It was a dark blue Donna Karan Couture suit that I got from the showroom in New York. Not that I'm highbrow or anything, but I had dated a girl who worked for the company. She got me the suit for almost nothing. Therefore, I made it my power suit, my interview suit.

When it was almost time for the car to take me to the station, I did something I had never done before. I had to put makeup on my hand because the white spot was so big it was noticeable. I didn't want to have to explain my disease in the midst of a job interview.

Luckily, the spot was on my left hand. I'm right handed. I could still shake hands and do what I needed to do, such as write. It was perfect.

It didn't really matter to me anyway, because as far as I

was concerned, this was just a stop along the way. I would keep this job just long enough to get my bearings straight and then I would head back to New York or Los Angeles.

I would also go to whatever doctor could cure this whole white spots thing. Then life for me would be right back on track.

It all sounded really simple.

On the other hand, I might not even like this place. And then I would just go back to my love in L.A. and spend the money I earned from Showtime. It would last me until I got another job. And judging by the looks of the newscast I was watching in my hotel room, unless the news director said something miraculous, I would just enjoy the free trip and go home, because that show was nothing to scream about.

A short time later, the Lincoln Town Car pulled through the gates of the station. The front of the building was old school TV. Its big white columns reminded me of how a government office would look down south. It wasn't quite plantation, but close enough to make me call my girlfriend and tell her to keep my side of the bed ready.

I try very hard not to judge something before I actually experience it. And something told me just to listen and make sure I got all of my questions answered. Sitting in the front lobby, I was ready for anything. I met the boss. Believe it or not, we actually hit it off immediately. He was a straight-talking New Yorker who used to work at my former station. That gave us a kinship from the start. I love NYC for the people. They are not afraid to shoot straight. That's the way it should be, even when it hurts. He didn't even give me a complete tour of the station. We talked in his office before going out to lunch to talk shop. Before we even sat down, I'd already decided to look for another job. And that was when my future boss said the one thing that started me thinking that this opportunity wouldn't be bad.

"First of all, forget that crap you saw this morning," he said. "We have a lot of work to do. We're getting a new set and a complete makeover." He had my attention.

From then on, the man proceeded to tell me everything I needed to hear to feel good about the job. The part I liked the most was the fact that he promised to allow me room to grow. He literally talked me into coming to Detroit right there at that table over an appetizer of calamari and a salmon entrée. Lucky for me, the only thing that seemed fishy was the meal.

On the way to the airport, I almost hadn't noticed that I never got to go to downtown Detroit. I never saw the heart of the city that I was to report on because the television station was in a nice suburb. I asked the driver if we could do a drive-by through downtown on the way to the airport.

"We have no time," he said.

Odd, but still if this was everything that the news director had just promised it could be, then this could be the opportunity of my life. On the other hand, he could be the best BS-er I'd ever met, and the city looked like crap, and I was about take a big bite of a chit sandwich.

I made no decisions or promises. I decided to go to L.A. and tell my girlfriend. We would decide together. Little did I know that this conversation would be the beginning of the end of my relationship. I did know that if she said to go, I would leave her, the relationship, and L.A. If she said she couldn't live without me, I would stay and make it work and learn to love her and myself the way we both deserved. This is one of those turning points in life. I was interested to see which way it was going to go.

Co Co's Bread and Biting Reality

"So, it's a three-year contract, and they want me to make the decision and get there as soon as possible."

This was the end of my explanation. We were sitting in my girl's favorite restaurant called Co Co's. It was just down the street from our apartment. Their dinner rolls that came complimentary with each meal were scrumptious. They melted in your mouth, even if it was wide open in a shocked position as you heard the cold, hard realities about your relationship. The bread was delicious. It was always fresh and hot, even if you were about to choke on it. After I explained my new job offer, I simply said, "I need to know how you feel about it. What do you think I should do?"

She paused for a few seconds, and then looked me in the eyes and said, "I think you should take it."

"What?" I said, as I struggled to keep it together.

"I think you should go."

I really didn't hear anything after that. It's weird how your brain shuts off any other input when you hear certain things like "There's no cure," and "I think you should take it." I guess it just fades into the background while your own thoughts race around the continuous track in your mind.

I was crushed. What did that mean? It didn't matter. I couldn't pack my stuff and get out of there fast enough. I wondered what love really was about. If she wanted me to go, did she still love me? It was all too confusing.

So I told my agent I would take the job.

He got back to me quickly with, "You start in two weeks." Wow, how quickly life can change. I had wanted to take six months between jobs in L.A. to find myself and my love, while charting a new path in my profession. It ended up being two months and one cool job.

A confusing relationship ended just before a three-year contract began in Detroit.

I was twenty-nine, and life was throwing me some curve balls that I couldn't seem to hit or even catch. New white spots were appearing on my hands, on my elbow, even on the inside of my nose. But I could still smell a big change coming.

FOUR

Lost and Found

A KID WAS SITTING ON THE FLOOR, playing with a toy car that he was driving up and down his mom's leg. It seemed like this little guy didn't have a worry in the world. And the mom was peacefully reading a book, just happy to know that her son was by her side. She didn't even look, but she knew he was there. It's funny how a mom can show love without moving an inch. Just by being a racetrack to a bored kid. When you're little, it seems like Mom is always in the right place at the right time.

At that moment, I would have killed to have my mom's leg to drive on. Mom is always the person to go to when times are hard. And moms always have something in their purse for you to play with or eat. She always has something to do when you're in an airport. And that's where I was, just sitting there watching people come and go.

I thought about that certain emotion that comes with traveling.

The airport is one of those places that's full of people with purpose. There's the "Hurry up, we're late!" people. They're mixed with the "Where is the restroom?" guys. And you can't forget the "Give me some tongue, I'm about to leave" couple. Then there's my favorite, the "My leg fell asleep! Get my medication!" grandma, who forgets all of it right when the grandkids show up.

All motivated by pure emotion. And I had a front row seat at the crossroads of love and family, work and home, everything that travel brings. The airport is also one of those common places where people are very different. Different languages, different clothing ... man, they even smell different.

But in the airport, people are also all strangely the same.

People who would never cross paths in life all have something in common in this place—they just want to get there. Get to their love/family/home. Get back to their lives. This crush of humanity was fun to watch. It made me feel like I was part of something, especially since I had nowhere to go. Remember, this was before 9/11. I didn't have a ticket.

I didn't have a flight that day, even though I asked Spirit Air how much a ticket from Detroit to L.A. would cost. I didn't have a reservation. Man, I didn't even have a plan. I had just gone to the airport because it was the only place I had to go.

I wanted to feel like I had something to do or somewhere I could go. So I went to the airport. I don't know if I even intended to buy a ticket or get a flight. I was just at the airport, watching people who did have somewhere to go and something to do, hoping that it would rub off on me.

I felt like I had no life in Detroit. I had just screwed up on the air (more on that later). I didn't have any friends or family in this new city. And I had nowhere to turn. So I *think* I went to airport with the intention of leaving. But when I got there I realized I had nowhere to go. As my oldest brother would say, "Ain't that a bitch."

I just sat there. I thought about life and watched other people busily going about their lives. Then I got all choked up. I could have cried … until I saw that kid playing with the car and the mom seemingly not paying attention to him.

It was simple, but it gave me comfort. I knew that my mother was not right there with me and she was not paying me any attention right now, but I was loved. It simplified everything in an instant. And watching the kid drive and have so much fun with the imaginary track on his mom's leg and foot made me happy. So, I sat and watched the families and the love and the basic need for togetherness being fulfilled. After about two hours of sitting and observing and regaining my perspective on life, I returned to my corporate-issued apartment. Meanwhile, I reached some crucial conclusions. My relationship with my girl in Los Angeles was over. There was no need to go to L.A. I would go back home to Mom in Washington, D.C., or to my sister's house in Las Vegas. I had just messed up on the television so badly that I was afraid to go into work the next day.

No!

Even with these weighty issues as my inventory, I decided right then and there at the airport that I was not going anywhere. No more running away.

All of this movement in the airport was about one thing: Everyone was rushing to get home. The solution to my angst, I realized, was simple: I needed to build a home of my own. I had chosen this new, struggling city as my home and I was going to make it work. I wasn't even sure what that meant, but I would try. I also didn't really know what to do, but leaving wasn't an option.

So, I got in my rental car and drove back to my apartment where I could stay for another twenty-three days. All I owned in the place was my clothing and my computer. But I made it feel like home by doing something that always makes me feel like I'm home, no matter where I am. I put on my favorite sweatshirt and started writing.

Writing soothes the soul. Especially when the first words I wrote in my journal were: *"I'm not going anywhere!!!"*

Picture Not Perfect

OK, so let's get to what happened at work that took me to the airport on that landmark day. To tell the truth to myself and to you, it wasn't just one thing that started me on the path of confusion. The job here in Detroit has become the job of my dreams, but it was far from that at first.

It's my job to be on TV and to shine light on people, places, and things that are interesting and entertaining. I don't report on death and destruction. I get to be the good news guy. I have an opportunity to let people know that the news can also be about the fun side of the human experience.

It's about sharing in each other ... but my methods of doing that are far from traditional. I call it controlled chaos. I do a lot of live TV, and I try not to pre-interview people too much or set up the scene too deliberately. I just let things happen, knowing that my communication skills will find a way to make the situation entertaining and/or compelling to watch.

The elements of surprise and spontaneity always enhance the entertainment event or person that I'm highlighting. Sometimes I'm not involved at all and the story is compelling. Other times, I need to infuse some new element that helps engage the fun for the television audience and the subject. I've been doing this for years. I don't cross the line, but it is spontaneous, unpredictable fun—the way live TV *should* be.

Now, Detroit is a news town. It's a hard city with lots of the stuff that hard news is all about: fires, murders, big business, and big government. It's a sports town with all of the major teams: the Lions of the National Football League, the Tigers of Major League Baseball, the National Basketball Association's Detroit Pistons, and we even have a darn good hockey team with the National Hockey League's Red Wings. Make no mistake: Detroit sports fans are passionate with a capital P.

With all that said, when I first arrived here in the Motor City, I don't think this city had ever seen a newscast with a reporter like me. I walked a high wire with the Flying Wallendas in the circus. I sang back-up on a live recording. I traded jobs with viewers. I featured a couple who had been married for fifty years. I did the good news in a fun way.

And the public was all in from the very beginning. Since arriving in Detroit, I've been greeted with open arms—from the public. But at work, not so. From the first day I was put on the air, the reception from my coworkers was cold to say the least. During my first week, the man who hired me seemed happy. So did everyone else, as long as he was around. Management even displayed my picture in the main hallway of the television station, along with portraits of the other anchors, right outside the big boss's office.

"Nice," I thought. "This job is going to go well. They saw this crazy stuff on my tape and they are behind me 100 percent. Good! I will work hard and leave my mark on this city." But then came my second week. I was strolling down the hall, minding my own business, when I looked up and noticed ...

They took my picture off the wall. It was gone. This change happened to occur just after my first live shot in the field. I was covering a tailgating party at a University of Michigan football game. It was the big interstate rivalry with Ohio. I did my thing, joked with a chef at a cookout, played catch with fellow tailgaters, and I even had two kids sing the different teams' fight songs. It was crazy and a little unpredictable, but good TV. At least, I thought it was. So I called back to the station to asked my producer, "How was that?"

The silence on the line was deafening. "OK," the producer finally said. "It was ... interesting."

Back at the station, one of the camera operators said, "Are you always so ... you know ... "

"Yep."

The chill intensified inside the studio. I did not feel comfortable on the set next to the other anchor. I don't think she liked my style. And I think my spontaneous approach made her uncomfortable. Our newscast together was rocky. I felt like my strength was in the field. So, after two painful shows, the news director pulled me off the desk and sent me back in the field.

The female anchor remained in the studio while I was live on location every weekend. It was actually a lot of fun, but the damage was done. The picture was off the wall, and the sting of failure was in the air.

So after about a month of struggle and a public dressing-down, I felt like an outcast. I had no family in this new city. I had nowhere to go and hang out. No one was giving any feedback or support except the guy who hired me. And by the way, my picture being down off the wall was a signal that was not to be ignored.

Back to the terminal (*not* a comment on the state of my career ... the *airport* terminal). I was there with nowhere else to turn, with nothing else to do, I felt had to do something or go somewhere. The airport was the perfect choice. I was going to get canned, and I would end up there anyway. So, I went to get comfortable before the actual event of my career's demise.

If the picture thing was any indication, my days were numbered. Plus, the white patches on my skin were getting larger. No matter what I did, they kept coming. Another had appeared on my scalp, and the inside of my nose continued to change as well. Did that mean it could get on my face? How dare this stuff get close to my face! I could be in some real trouble if this spread any further.

Part of me wanted to just leave and turn white on my own, rather than have it happen on television in front of thousands of strangers. But I didn't know where to go and hide. And I was afraid of failing. I was even more terrified that I would eventually turn completely white.

I felt like an out-of-control train going down the wrong track. There was no conductor in the engine room. And a broken track loomed ahead.

I wasn't just afraid. I was mortified.

Staying Power

I had begun writing in a journal while in New York. I had started writing a one-man show for myself. That inspired me so much that I began to compose the script with the intention of someday performing it as a stage play.

This creativity gave me inspiration and focus. It took me away from my old friend, the ceiling. Writing in the journal and composing the script filled me with excitement and happiness. And my writing blessed me with something that television had almost beaten out of me: hopes and dreams.

So outside of my Detroit TV job, I indulged my passion by working on that script and writing in the journals that I had begun in New York.

At the time, I didn't even know that it was called journaling. I simply bought a marble-colored looseleaf book and started writing in it. I would jot down my ideas for segments on the news, treatments for TV shows, jokes, and funny stories that would happen to me. It was all about my thoughts, my dreams, and everything in between.

I loved the way it felt to tell someone this stuff—even though the someone I was telling was me. I just kept on writing. I never really told anyone about it because a part of me thought that it was girlie. But more and more, I found myself lost in the pages of my own thoughts. Writing and reading them was—and still is—a cathartic experience. It liberates my mind and frees my heart. Through writing, I finally found my home. And it was inside me the whole time.

By "finding myself," I discovered answers to some of my most vexing questions. It started at the airport, when I decided to make a stand. No more leaving! I had to stay until I became the man I want to be in every way.

I want a cure for this disease. I want to be great at all aspects of my job. I want to find the love of my life. And I will stay in Detroit as long as it takes to find it all. I made a pledge that night to find myself. To find that little kid in me who was sitting on the floor playing with his mom's leg and enjoying life without running away.

I summoned every ounce of courage in my soul and decided to stay, no matter what.

To do that, I would have to utilize another talent: my acting skills. Now, I have always been a fan of acting. Even though I had been performing since the age of seven, it was not my dream to be a famous star in Hollywood. My dream was to live and work in New York as a performer. And then my plan evolved into becoming a television host. I wanted to do both in New York City. I thought that was where the real professional performers lived.

As I composed my play and wrote in my journal, my writing inspired me to dream. It also gave me the time to step out of myself and apply some of my acting training to what I do in broadcasting. I was so confident in my abilities to ad-lib that I never thought I wasn't good at everything else. I must have been good or I wouldn't have gotten this far. But as I analyzed my craft from different angles, I broke it down to the basics, the same way I would evaluate a character in a script. I examined my history in the business. I looked at the context and experience that each of my previous jobs had afforded me.

While I've always been able to perform, broadcast journalism is ten percent performance and ninety percent hard work and research. Suddenly I realized I had always been so focused on performance that I didn't see the truth of the profession. I was great at live TV. And I had developed into a good, solid writer. But I really needed some work in other areas.

Specifically, I needed to focus on the way I gathered and reported hard news, both in the field and in the studio. Because confidence wasn't going to cover up the fact that I was uncomfortable with harder stories. It was not my background. And no matter how I wanted to be the master of all TV broadcasting, my history was in the coverage and delivery of entertainment news. I needed to revisit the basics of electronic newsgathering if I wanted to go forward. This was a sobering realization. Not only would I stay and pursue my best health and happiness, but I would also work hard to correct my professional shortcomings. All while dealing with a disease that was making me turn white in a city where I had no family and no close friends.

Whew! When I left the airport, I vowed not to leave this place until I was great at every aspect of my job. I would not run to my agent to find the next job. It was time to put in some hard work. And yes, I would stumble. But with each fall, I would get up, brush myself off, analyze why it happened, understand my mistake, and work hard to correct it. I would go all the way back to the basics and use this job as my opportunity to grow. I pledged to invest in me. All the while, I marveled at the irony of my situation.

There I was, vowing to be my best on live TV, as my body was turning white. Of all the diseases that a black man working in television could get, I got this thing that is so visual and so shocking. I thought the Almighty was sending me a message and it might be time for me to listen.

As a result, that trip to the airport started me off on the best journey of my life—and I never even got on a plane. But looking back I can say that it's been a beautiful ride. Many times, I wasn't sure where I was going. Along the way, I have soared and crashed. But I wouldn't change anything. And I mean anything. That trip to the airport changed my life. It was the real beginning of my life journey. And it didn't cost me a thing.

I have found my dreams, my family, and my fears. I have become the man I always wanted to be.

The Adventure Begins

I like wearing a tuxedo. Something about it makes you feel sophisticated, even if you're flicking peas across the plate in a game of "closest to the fork." That's a fun way to pass the time at long award shows and banquets. Until your category comes up, that is. Then you forget all about the tux and the food because your nerves kick into overdrive. I was sitting at the table in this elegant hotel ballroom, feeling as nervous as the first time I went "parking" with a girl in high school.

The local Emmy Awards program meant much more than kissing in the car. It was the recognition and celebration that my work was outstanding in broadcast journalism. I was nominated for two Emmys. And one of my categories was second on the list of awards to be given out. So my cameraman and I were nervously thrilled to be in the company of some of the beloved and respected veteran journalists from the Detroit media market. It was an incredible honor to be nominated in the same category as Erik Smith from ABC affiliate Channel 7. He's won more Emmys than I have birthdays, but I believed I still had a chance.

Finally, the emcee spoke: "And the Emmy goes to 'scooter story,' Lee Thomas, Fox 2 News!" It was a report where I took a new electrically motorized scooter to a local university to let the students test the product and give it the thumbs up or thumbs down. My cameraman and I thought the story turned out well—and I guess the Emmy board agreed.

That's right, people! I had just won an Emmy! This man who was once a little five-year-old boy standing in front of the TV declaring that he would grow up and devote his career to television had just won the top honor in his field! As I rose from the seat and the audience applauded, I marveled at the fact that my secret airport drama—when I almost made a run for it—occurred only eighteen months prior to this pinnacle moment.

It felt surreal. And bittersweet.

Don't get me wrong; I loved the fact that I was now an award-winning journalist. But on my way up to the podium to accept the first of four Emmys I would win here in Detroit— during what should be and was one of the happiest moments of my life—I was trying to hide my left hand.

I didn't put makeup on it. And the white spot had become much bigger. Plus, I had some new spots on my scalp, on my hand, and my torso. To hide my new whiteness, I grew my hair longer. Clothing covered my torso.

But the hand was spotted white for all to see. And every news executive in town would see my secret. Maybe it would cause them not to hire a black man who was turning white.

If you're thinking this is being paranoid, don't. About

one month earlier, a local company that was a major supplier to Detroit's huge auto industry had called me to host their internal training video. It's one of the many side jobs that TV people can take to supplement their income. And those side jobs, by the way, can become lucrative. Especially this one.

The company's CEO called a talent agent who offered me a payment figure that I couldn't refuse. The meeting was scheduled for my day off. Have I mentioned that I usually don't wear makeup on my days off? So for the interview, I put on my suit and got all made up—except for the left hand. I decided not to put makeup there, just to hold onto *part* of my day off. But interviewing for a potential job is just like going to work on your day off. You have to take a shower and wear a suit. It was work. When I arrived, the CEO was friendly enough. In his mid- to late-fifties, he couldn't say enough about how he loved what I do on TV. He said my youthful approach was perfect to keep his employees interested in this internal training video. He even gave me a tour of the facility.

All of that would have been great if he hadn't spent seventy-five percent of the conversation looking at—or trying not to have me catch him looking at—*my hand*. The CEO couldn't stop staring. When he thought I wasn't looking, of course. You know, I would look away for a second; he'd look at my hand. Then, when I'd look back, he'd look away.

After a while, it became a game to me, like a tennis match. He would volley a look when I was off guard and I would quickly spin and try to catch him. But he was the Pete Sampras of glances. I never brought up the subject of my hand. Neither did he.

The meeting, or should I say the match, went well. The hosting job would have been the kind I like—easy and fun. I left thinking I may get this job all the way up until I raised my right hand to shake his hand. He was very apprehensive and all but pulled away. I know he went and washed his hands right after. I never heard from that guy again.

Later that week, the agent said the CEO changed his mind. "He just decided to go in a different direction," the agent said.

That's the show biz way of saying "no." That incident flashed through my thoughts as I headed up to the podium at the Emmy Award ceremony.

Standing before the movers and shakers of my industry to accept my trophy, I felt almost naked. I felt vulnerable. I felt like I had no chance that other TV executives would hire me now. They had seen my hand. And like the CEO of that company, they would pull away in secret revulsion with a half-handshake.

Joy and sadness overwhelmed me all at once. Was everyone in the room looking at my Emmy, my beaming smile, or my hand? Either way, I stood triumphant with a prestigious award in hand. This Emmy symbolized my commitment to working hard to become a better journalist. By conquering my career conundrum, I had honored the pledge I had made while watching the little boy in the airport. I had grown up, faced my problems head-on, and now I was being rewarded for that effort. Somehow, I would do the same with my other challenges.

While the exuberance of the moment filled me with confidence that my future would sparkle with success, it again tasted bittersweet. Because I knew that the real fight was about to begin. Backstage, as I gripped the Emmy in my right hand and glanced at the white spot on my left hand, I made yet another vow to myself:

I will win this fight!

I will take it as far as necessary to win.

I will be whole again, or die trying.

I will stop this disease from turning me white. Period.

I would go to whatever doctor could help me on any continent. Nothing would stop me. And I finished my personal pledge with the words of one of my favorite fictional characters, Forrest Gump:

"That's all I have to say about that."

Halle Can't See Me Like This

It was July 2004, and I was sitting outside the interview room for one of the biggest stars on the planet. Some people would say that she is the most beautiful woman alive. I completely agree with that assessment. I was waiting for my turn to interview Ms. Halle Berry. A steady stream of reporters filed from the room that was packed with cameras, publicists, makeup and hair artists, and the woman that men all over the world dream about.

Meanwhile, guess what was on my mind? Nope, I was not thinking about my questions. Having interviewed celebrities for more than a decade, I was not nervous about meeting her. In fact, I had talked with her before. It's my job.

No, at this moment when any man on the planet would be excited beyond words to sit face-to-face with Halle Berry … my singular thought was about my hands. What will she do when she sees my hands? Would it be a look of concern for herself … fearing that what I have is contagious? Then she would hesitate to shake my hand. Would it be a look of sympathy? That would make me feel like anything but a whole, handsome man. Or would she even see me? She could get so transfixed by my hands that she would never look up at my face.

All of the above reactions have occurred as I've interviewed different celebrities. I've even heard some of them mumble comments as I'm leaving the room when they think I can't hear them anymore.

What would Ms. Berry do? And why did it bother me so much?

Now, don't get me wrong, at that moment I felt happier than I ever had professionally. I had made a great name for myself in the business and in Detroit. I love my job. Over the years with every challenge I faced, I seemed to have found a way to grow and improve. I've made this job, *the job*. I'm in the middle of my third contract with just over seven years at the station. The job has evolved over the years as I have evolved.

At this point in my career, I am an entertainment reporter and field anchor for Fox 2 News in Detroit. I'm live on the morning show, either in the studio with the anchors or out on location. I do a great job at both. On my beat, I keep viewers up on the latest movies, TV shows, and Hollywood stuff. Plus, I get to cover all of the events and people profiles that I want. And those quirky little stories that make you smile. I also do an "On The Road" segment with an RV and my cameraman; we tour around Michigan finding hidden treasures. This is it for me. I have found a way to make this job my dream job. The next thing is to have my own talk show, but if that happens or not, I'm very happy with my job.

But sitting outside Halle Berry's interview room, I pondered one thing that I have yet to figure out: The vitiligo is perplexing and slightly menacing—and no matter what expert I go to and no matter what I seem to try, things just keep getting worse. I'm turning white and Halle Berry would see it the moment I walked into the room. At that point, my hands were more white than brown. But even more disturbing, white spots started to appear on my face. I covered them with makeup. But the hands were too hard to cover. And when I did cover them, the makeup would come off all over my clothes.

You can only imagine the different parts of your body that your hands touch regularly. Well, with makeup on my hands, every time I touch anything, and I mean any part of my body, a little brown mark gets left behind.

Since I am a brown man, it looks like dirt. So did I want Halle to think I was dirty or diseased? Believe it or not, it was a tough call, but I went with the truth—diseased. Therefore I chose not the put makeup on my hands. She would see a black man with white hands.

I still don't know why it mattered so much. Why did Halle noticing my vitiligo bother me? She probably wouldn't even say anything about it. But then again, what if she did?

"Lee Thomas, Fox 2 Detroit," a young lady announced as

I entered the interview room. Walking toward the reporter's chair, which faces the star in her seat, I exchanged hellos with some of the crew members whom I've met on previous stories. Before I even got to the chair, Halle spoke: "Haven't we spoken before?" She looked me straight in the eyes. "Yes, we have," I said. "I'm flattered that you remember me."

She remembered me! Halle Berry remembered me!

She was as gracious as ever, even though the movie she was promoting, *Catwoman*, was not so good. In fact, according to the "Razzies" (The Golden Raspberry Award Foundation) it was the worst film of the year. But it was a great interview. And if she noticed my hands or not, I had no idea. She is a gracious and beautiful woman. And I think that's what makes her such a big star. It's real.

Now you might think Halle Berry remembering me would be the highlight of my day. Any man in his right mind would be on a cloud. It would be the feather in your cap, not only for that day, but for much longer.

But that was not what I was thinking about as I left the room. Did she remember me for me, or is it because of my hands? They are hard to forget since they are almost completely white. I couldn't shake it. I guess the reason that this bothers me so much is because I seem to have found my dream, and this thing that is beyond my control may be the only thing that people remember about me. And it just may, at some point, be the reason that my dream gets deferred. Because yes, she saw my hands, but what she couldn't see were the spots on my face and neck ... or the spots this has left on my heart and mind.

When I look at myself in the mirror, it's getting harder to see me.

Monster Me

Journal entry: November 14, 2004

> *I look into the face of this monstrous mutation of my beautiful brown skin. It is being devoured by this void of white that is slowly stealing me from myself. The old me would talk to almost any woman I wanted. Now, I don't even go out. I'm a prisoner of this disease. I'm trapped. And Halle would have to miss out on her future husband because of it. Halle Berry represented every woman that I talked myself out of approaching because they would never fall for a guy who's turning white.*
>
> *Now in my mind, vitiligo is the thing that's holding me hostage and I can't do anything to get out. I know who I am on the inside; I am the man I always wanted to be. But my exterior terrifies me. Afraid to live, afraid to love, afraid to be comfortable in my own skin. The thing about conquering*

New York and finding my way in the world of broadcasting is very distant and insignificant compared to losing myself. I don't know if finding me has anything to do with a cure. But I know that I want this feeling of inadequacy to go away. And even more important, I want to live without struggling to decide if I want to go out without makeup. And when I do go out I have to be prepared to deal with any situation like the people who walk up and say, "You look kinda like that guy on TV. You're not him, are you?" Now that's a great pointed question usually followed by, "What happened to you?"

So, after speaking with the most beautiful woman in the world, I don't know if I will ever find love or myself or my life again. I know that I will give it everything I have and go to the end of the Earth and back to find something that is much more important than a cure. I need to find my peace of mind.

I still didn't know the lesson in this disease. But I knew the real fight had just begun.

Two Little Girls

The skin on my face is softer than it's ever been. I used to have acne; now it's all gone. In theory, I fit the flattering description of "tall, dark, and handsome." The tall and the handsome are definitely arguable points of taste. And the dark is very much in question.

The amount of white on my face is amazing. It's hard to see me anymore. This is bad. Would you ever think that this is the face of a four-time Emmy-winning television journalist? This is the face of a guy who goes to work in the public eye, only to return home and then debate the pluses and minuses of going to the mall. Sometimes that debate resulted in a decision not to go out of the house the entire weekend. So many times, I thought I should just quit and go hide somewhere. Other times, I just hid out. There are times of weakness. But I have vowed to stay engaged in life no matter what. I had no idea "what" would mean watching myself turn white. I never envisioned this. I call it the phobia of me. I look like a monster.

I've recently come to a brand-new conclusion that is just plain weird: I've become afraid of small children! It's not the snot or the coughing. It's not the loud play or the infinite energy. I actually love kids. They are the most honest people on the planet. And that's where the fear begins. Their honesty can put me in awkward situations. Because they say things that leave me speechless and embarrassed, standing mute in a crowd of gawkers.

Imagine dozens of children. They were loud and happy

and full of life. Blonde-, brown-, and black-haired bundles of energy and honesty. Their eyes were bright, and they were ready to do what all kids are eager to do: Play! Lucky for them, they were about to test-drive what was supposed to be the safest, most kid-friendly new playscape. It would be the prototype for playscapes of the future. And I was there to report on the future of frolic. It was one of those feature reports I look forward to because kids are fun and unpredictable.

For the story, we brought a whole group of kids to test the playscape and see if the company's predicted future for this new product was real. Or at least to see if all of the PR people for the company were accurate in their assessment. As the kids were getting off the bus and heading into the building, I was certain that they could not see the white spots on my face. My makeup does an excellent job of making my whole face appear naturally brown.

But the kids could see the spots on my hand. As they romped off the bus and into the play area that we had designated to shoot the story, the teacher said, "This is Mr. Thomas. He is a reporter." Now, these kids were little. Preschoolers, ages three to about five. When they looked at me, their reactions were mixed. Some pointed. A few looked a little scared. Others even laughed. They're kids, I could deal with it. Then I saw one golden-haired little angel who wasn't really paying attention. And as she turned around to see what all of the other kids were looking at, she almost bumped right into me. Teetering, she was about to take a tumble. Now, I'm six foot two inches tall and huge compared to a little one like her. I extended my hand to stop her from falling. She looked up, stared at my hand ... and burst into tears! Horror distorted her face as she stood, paralyzed with fear, bawling. This little angel was petrified of me. And I didn't know what to do. I stood frozen in momentary shock.

I was sorry. I wanted to hug her or help her. But she ran to the teacher. She ran from my hands. I was dumbfounded. The teacher distracted the child and soothed her fears and her tears. The adults stared for a short eternity. Then they did what we all do best—act like nothing happened and ignore the situation in the hope that time will make it disappear. No one said a thing to me about what had happened, ever. Instead, after an awkward moment of silence, we all got back to work. As I went through the motions of the story, my insides were full of sadness and shock. I scared a child just by reaching out my hands! What if the little girl had seen my face!

I finished my job and the shoot went well, but the story left a much bigger impression on me than I'm sure that report did on the viewers. I retreated to the solitude of my house for several weekends. I refused to go out in public without makeup on my face. I didn't want to scare children or feel like a helpless spectacle. I didn't want the pity. But I promised myself never to wear makeup when I was not at work. So, I just didn't go anywhere, except to work and back home. That became my routine for a while. I would get my groceries right after work, so I still had on makeup. I would not accept speaking engagements on the weekends, because I really didn't want to put on the makeup. I was in a self-imposed prison, because I was scaring children. Try and get your head around that. I couldn't.

After a while, I started going out again, without makeup. This was my way of slowly blending back into a normal life. I know you can't hide forever, but you can take a break to regain strength. And I had. But I limited my excursions to places where people were used to seeing me: My gym, my favorite health food restaurant, my grocery store.

During one quick trip to the store, wearing no makeup, I was perusing the soup aisles.

Let's see, I had already gotten some minestrone soup from the top shelf. It is my favorite organic blend besides tomato soup. Next from aisle number two was the rice cakes. The ranch flavor are my favorite. So now it was a quest for rice cakes. But I didn't see them. There they were, at the back of the bottom shelf. I got on my knees and reached back to find them. They are worth all this effort. Just as I stretched to obtain my treat, I looked up into the cutest brown eyes. I was suddenly face-to-face with the most adorable, concerned little face I had seen since my niece was a toddler.

This little girl was probably three years old. And she had something to say to me.

"Ooo got a boo-boo," she said with a voice that demanded a smile. And not only did she have her little brow wrinkled with concern, the little girl was reaching out to touch my face. And she did it without fear. She just extended her pudgy little hand, placed her fingertips on my cheek, and said it again.

"Ooo got a boo-boo."

I froze. Should I run? Stand up straight? Stay frozen and hope she doesn't run in fear? I just hoped she wouldn't cry.

As I started to stand, she actually reached out and touched me with her other hand.

"Does it hurrrreet?" she asked.

"What?" I said.

Mom translated: "She wants to know if it hurts."

She was asking me if I was hurt. What a big heart for such a little person! That little girl didn't know what a great thing she had just done for me. With one touch of her little hand, like a miracle worker, she had healed a grown man's pain. She just reached out to share in what she thought was my pain. But she actually reached out and without even trying, touched my heart.

Her mom just smiled and said, "Sarah, leave the man alone."

"It's OK," I said quickly. Then I told the child, "No, young lady, it doesn't hurt." I touched her on the head, then stood up. She stood there, just looking at me like she had more to say.

"It doesn't hurrrreet?"

"No, cutie. It doesn't hurt." I smiled at her. Confident that I was all right, she grinned and said, "OK." With that, she was off to continue her exploration of the fascinating world of the supermarket. It was like she was not afraid because I was not in pain.

I doubt the little girl or her mom realized what had just happened, but that little hand and that big heart dramatically transformed my outlook about going out in public. Right there in Holiday Market, down from the bread and Wheat Thins, next to the rice cakes and soup, I regained my freedom. I found myself comfortable outside in public again without any cover.

That day changed me. How could someone so little and innocent have helped me so much? The innocence of children is golden and they speak nothing but the truth. They don't have a filter.

Both little girls helped me to understand myself. They

helped me to clarify what I call the duality of me. They exhibited the two extremes of reactions that I get every day—plus everything in between—in relation to how people feel about seeing me with this shocking, visual disease.

One reaction was based on ignorance. And that's not a negative thing. The little girl had never seen anything like me before; sometimes ignorance can cause fear. But the other little girl in the grocery store thought she knew what was wrong. Because of that, she had no fear. She had compassion and concern and displayed a kind heart.

Since then, as this disease has worsened, I've gotten many kinds of reactions from children and adults. Some are unaffected. Some can't look away. Still others just can't look me in the eyes. I understand them all and embrace their humanity. Because to be honest, sometimes *I* want to scream when I see myself in the mirror. *I* want to cry until it's all better. Other times, I don't even notice it because my mind is somewhere else.

From the innocence of children I've found my understanding. And I want to give thanks to the two little girls who will probably never even remember meeting me. Two young ladies who changed me forever. They freed me and helped me to understand myself more then they will ever know.

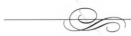

FIVE

Medical Mystery Tour

"ARE YOU READY?"

"Yes, How much time to I get today?"

"You're almost up to the limit."

"Well, I'm buttered and ready. Put me on bake at 350."

It was like an oven, but when I cooked, it seemed like I would never be done. One of the many treatments for vitiligo is to put on some cream and stand in an ultraviolet light. This light can damage the skin, so you have to start off with short segments of light that gradually build until you reach the maximum of about twelve minutes.

The treatment requires the application of a medicated cream fifteen minutes before entering the light booth. Then you stand in the ultraviolet light to stimulate your pigment. When you start off, you are in the light for only a few seconds. But if you go as prescribed, three times a week, your time increases. I was up to about ten minutes.

I began these treatments after finding the best doctor in the Midwest. This physician had successfully treated many patients. He and his staff were very nice and accommodating. We tried all kinds of light spectrums and lasers; since he was on the cutting edge, he would get some treatments that were still in the testing phase. He would test them on me. Still, the vitiligo would not let go.

It's still here, and I'm still fighting vitiligo with all that I currently know how. I have found a medical doctor who's a "naturalpathic" doctor, and we have come up with a regimen of treatment. I am hopeful for results.

All of the emotion from the Emmys was great and it propelled me into a medical search and research mode like I have never been in before. I applied creams and stood in ultraviolet light. And I tried every laser and light and steroid treatment that was the latest and the greatest. During one eighteen-month period, I slathered on the cream, then stood in a lighted box three times a week.

I did experience light pigment regeneration, but if I missed some treatments, the pigment would fade. Even worse, the new color would come in darker, while more white patches would appear. This method of treatment—treating the spots rather than the *cause* of the spots—forced me to draw a very important conclusion on my own: Conventional doctors are not really concerned with the cause of this disease. They just wanted to make the pigment come back. It wasn't making sense to me. They don't know what causes it, but they have all of these different and expensive treatments that *should* fix the problem. Why? According to statistics, these treatments work for more than sixty percent of vitiligo patients. That sounded great every time I heard it.

But one major problem remained: This stuff wasn't working on me!

After more than six years of trying doctors and treatments, I was fed up. The last three of the seven were very intense and involved light treatments that were starting to harden my skin. It was time to ask myself, "How far will you go to get the results that you want?" My answer was clear.

I would apply the same indomitable spirit to my health quest as I had to my professional life. I would view every mistake or problem as great opportunities to learn and acquire new knowledge.

The lesson that you learn from these experiences is like a crash course that educates you and brings you closer to your ultimate goal. This philosophy is one of those life lessons that I would never compromise.

I wasn't giving up on doctors or conventional medicine. But I would start keeping my own files and ask more in-depth questions. I would do whatever it takes to educate myself and understand as much as I can about this disorder. I would also try a holistic approach at the same time. I would keep trying until I got results.

When I get those results, I will build on them until the goal is complete. That may sound crazy to a lot of people. I'm not saying I know more than any medical professional. I just need to do as much as I can without giving up. Ever!

This road will be tough. And expensive. My insurance is not covering all of the cost. So I am paying for a lot of this myself. And when I'm paying, I'll ask as many questions as I want. I'll tape the conversations if I want. I don't know what this new level of commitment means. It may take years, but I can't think of a better way to spend my time. And with that as my premise, the answer to how far I would go was clear.

As far as I need to go to achieve my goal.

Little did I know how many years or how many different kinds of doctors and treatment regimens I would—and continue to—encounter.

History Is No Mystery

Some people believe in reincarnation.

I don't. But I do believe we are the product of our heritage, and that in itself is a form of reincarnation. The people who made you and raised you gave you a set of beliefs. They explained your world to you. They taught you how to walk. They taught you how to talk.

And this is even bigger and more important: They taught you how and what to eat.

The quest to cure my body of disease has forced me to examine my eating habits. I discovered that my childhood diet virtually set the stage in my body for disease to play a starring role, as it does for the millions of Americans who suffer from a plethora of diet-related illnesses such as diabetes, colon cancer, hypertension, obesity, and on and on.

I share this not to blame or shame myself or my family; they were doing the best they knew how to do at the time. And we were not unlike thousands of other families—especially African-American families. Since my mother came from South Carolina, she served traditional soul food. Chitlins, a lot of fried chicken, biscuits and gravy, and bread with butter were mainstays on the Thomas family's dinner table. With my dad as an officer in the military stationed in Fort Sill, Oklahoma, and Mom staying home to take care of us kids, her home-cooked meals were like mother-love on a plate. Every bite was nourishing to the heart and soul for me, my three brothers, and my two sisters.

My favorite meal? Pancakes swimming in syrup and butter. Sometimes I would eat that low-fiber, sugary delight for breakfast, lunch, and dinner! I also chowed on grits with cheese, butter, and bacon mixed in! Yum! What about fruits and vegetables? I wasn't too keen on either. The closest I came to fruit was the artificial grape flavoring in the several glasses of Kool-Aid that I drank every day. It was fun to make. And when I poured that packet of purple flavoring into the jar to mix it with water, I added mounds of sugar. It was more like Kool-Aid syrup. At school, my favorite beverage was Mountain Dew, which washed down my lunch of Doritos and Twinkies. Seriously, that was my mid-day meal in high school.

Today, with the hindsight of two decades and the knowledge of a nutritionist, I realize I was never taught basic nutrition. Or how healthy eating can prevent illness, while a crappy diet invites disease.

Unfortunately, when your family taught you what and how to eat, it may not have been a conscious choice, but you learn by watching and listening and tasting. These impressions were not just in what they said; their actions made the most powerful impact.

These create the blueprint for your life. My illness has inspired me to analyze the blueprint of my life. It has forced me to examine the "big picture" of my life, my family, and our culture in order to comprehend all the factors that put me in this physical and emotional place today.

What I've learned is that every culture, ethnicity, and individual has a history. It's the knowledge that you learn from the moment you are conscious through your pre-teen years. Those lessons—from listening to music in the womb, or hearing parents yell, or receiving no attention, or even being raised by the television—create your core beliefs and responses. All of this occurs in the unconscious mind.

For example, when I was a child, I had the feeling that I would be in front of many people. I believed it even before I knew what it meant. I also loved my family and was a naturally happy child. In fact, I was the kind of kid who would stand in line at the store with my mother and sing a song and dance to entertain myself and anybody else who wanted to watch. I was pure joy. But when I was three, the negative vibes of the world started to shut down my happy spirit. I learned about the struggle of being black in America. Worse, I learned that I was supposed to accept that struggle. Now, this isn't about race. Everyone has different rules or restrictions placed on their lives at an early age, whether you are Jewish, Italian,

Russia, Indian, or another ethnic group. A blueprint exists for you and everyone. But how you choose to physicalize your pressures is unique to you.

Remember the butterflies in the stomach when you are standing next to a pretty girl or getting ready to speak in public? That is the physicalization of an emotion. But all of your emotions get translated into a physical state. And I think the bad ones can cause disease.

For me, when I was nervous or under pressure, I would stand straight and tense the muscles of my lower back. And that's where my back pain began. The lower back is connected to the colon, and the colon is your cleaning system. If it becomes impaired you don't get clean and then come your problems. Many of those problems begin with the standard American diet. It is just so *sad*. Add the temptations of fast food and our all-you-can-eat mentality, and we really don't stand a chance. By the time you are in your forties, you will have some kind of disease or ailment. And the standard African-American diet is even worse because it's based on scraps, leftovers, or slave food—the parts of the pig the "big house" threw out.

I'm not condemning my history or the American diet in general. What I am blaming is the amounts we choose to eat. That is the problem, and over time it can cripple and kill you.

Or in my case, turn you white.

I want to make a very clear point right now. I'm not a doctor or a medical professional of any kind. But I do know that when I eat unhealthy food, I see new spots. The solution is to change your diet, and understand what parts of your historical blueprint contributed to the unhealthy way of life. Then you can change it. This is the formula for changing your physical being. But first you must comprehend the mental dimension of our human blueprints.

Whether your childhood was filled with love or hate, violence or nurturing, healthy habits or destructive ones, they all took root in your subconscious mind. And that is the place where your body and mind act without you. It's the part of your mind that tells your heart to pump, your lungs to breathe, your cells to accept nourishment. It's the part that makes you react before that first rational thought.

You may call it instinct or gut feeling, but it's the part of you that acts or reacts without you consciously telling your body to do anything. Sometimes you don't even understand why. This is the subconscious mind. But once you are aware of this subconscious, now you can understand yourself better. And you can reprogram some of those undesirable patterns. I personally started to reprogram myself in terms of my habit of negative thought avalanches and my terrible eating habits.

The Main Pain

"Scooby, Scooby Doo!"

"Scrappy, Scrappy Doo!"

They have solved the mystery again and my man—or should I say my dog—Scooby and his nephew, Scrappy, are off to help the gang solve another mystery. I always liked watching that cartoon. And just as I prepare to jump out of bed and yell, "Scrappy Doo!" a mystery of my own forces me to solve it.

First of all, Scrappy Doo is smart and cute. But nothing is cute or smart about the pain in my back. For a split-second, it slices like a knife through my lower back. The excruciating bolt doubles me over. I am stunned, unable to move or think until the pain subsides.

I fall back onto the bed until, just moments later, I can breathe and think and move once again.

The pain is gone for now. But I know it will be back.

These excruciating episodes happened enough times to convince me that something was very wrong. But, like my quest to determine the cause of my vitiligo, I never would have guessed how far I would go or how long it would take to find the answer to this back-aching mystery.

When it began years ago, I started going to a chiropractor. He worked with me for a year and a half. During that time, I realized a few things. First and foremost, this adjusting of the back thing was painful. In some positions, a pain throbbed continuously. As a result, I avoided those positions.

Adjusting my back didn't help, but the chiropractor did. After about eighteen months, he closed the curtain and said, "Your back is straight. You should go to an internal specialist. I think the pain you are experiencing is one of the organs in the same area."

I went to my regular doctor, who performed a battery of tests.

"I don't detect anything out of the ordinary," she said, "but this should ease the pain." She gave me painkillers! Without even understanding the cause of the pain, she prescribed pills. I didn't understand that, so I refused the medication.

Maybe it's the reporter in me, but I will not take anything unless I understand why and how it's going to help me. If I had taken the medication she gave me, it would have been like ignoring my body. My body sent me pain to tell me something was wrong. If I covered up the pain, I feared the problem would get worse and I wouldn't even know it.

I decided right there to go to another doctor and another doctor and another ... until I got an explanation I understood and a treatment I agreed with.

I consulted with an M.D. who had worked with many

professional athletes and was celebrated as one of the best back specialists around. "I don't see a problem with your back," he said, after looking at my chart. "I will give you some muscle relaxers and that should ease the pain. Have you ever gotten your internal organs checked?"

"No."

"Well, this may not be a back problem at all," the doctor said. "It could be something wrong with whatever organ is pressing against that part of your back."

That for me was a light bulb moment. So, I took his advice, but not the muscle relaxers. I didn't want a mask for the problem. I wanted a solution. And that sent me on another quest that has opened my eyes. After a couple more years of traditional doctors, I went the holistic route.

That was after listening to that gut feeling you get when you're scared or nervous. I was certain that my problems—and the answers—were literally lurking in my gut. And my instincts were confirmed by a medical doctor who was also a naturalpathic doctor. He ran several tests.

With the results in hand, he said something that I already suspected. But now it finally made sense. "There is a swelling in your colon," he said. "And it may have been there for years. It's probably the cause of your back problem and may be contributing to the vitiligo."

Bang! There was the answer I had been waiting for. The doctor explained how years of a bad diet wears away your intestinal flora. Those are the good and bad bacteria that help you digest food. After you wear them away to a certain point, you begin to have problems. It's like having your pipes clogged. Eventually they burst or have gunk in them that just makes your blood like the dirty oil that will eventually ruin an engine.

The bottom line was the swelling in my colon caused the pain; certain foods aggravated the pain. It also meant my colon was not absorbing the nutrients in food properly. I understood that, but I wanted to know even more. So I went to another specialist: a colon expert. Much to the doctor's surprise, I requested a colonoscopy—a surgical procedure in which the doctor inserts a tiny camera into the large intestine to examine the walls.

When the doctor agreed, I gave her a "high five." Then, like Scooby and Scrappy on a mission to find answers, I discovered mine.

Turns out, the bottom line of my medical journey is quite simple. The look inside my colon revealed the answer that made the most sense of all:

Crohn's disease. This chronic condition causes the colon walls to swell and even scab over, causing a variety of problems, especially that crippling back pain.

I am very thankful that I have an answer, no matter how long it took to find it. My next mystery: Is there a definite connection between vitiligo and Crohn's disease?

I don't know yet. But I do believe that I cannot just live with these problems. I can also conquer them. Maybe it sounds crazy, but solving this mystery has taken me to places I would have never gone. I have a healthier lifestyle and a better approach to a balanced diet than I've ever had in my life.

It has also put my reporting skills to excellent use, as I've dealt with doctors and the so-called medical "experts."

Remember, Scooby, Shaggy, and the gang never gave up— even when they found out the person they had trusted was the bad guy. So my Scooby approach to solving a medical problem is silly, but it works. The trick is to ask questions, even the ones you fear might sound stupid. It's your body, your health, and your responsibility. If your doctor responds in Scooby-speak with, "Rie ron't row," don't give up. Because the doctor may never say they don't know in a way you can understand. But if you ask enough questions, you will realize that your doctor may not know and it's time to get another opinion. So ask questions! And don't leave until you get an answer you understand.

That's where I am now. My journey is not over. I am still on my quest for answers. I will document my medical mystery tour so others may find an easier path one day.

Right now, I know how to manage my back pain—with my diet. Remember what your mother used to say: "You are what you eat" and "Eat those veggies!" And think about that ancient wise man, Hippocrates, who once said, "Let food be your medicine." Well, mother wit and the ancient Greek guy are having a huge influence on my wellness plan. It's all about what I eat, and it works!

After years of research and adventurous quests to clinics across the country, I've devised a vegetable-based diet that is giving my body what it needs to heal. It is a radical change from the processed, salty, sugary, high-fat foods in the meat-based diet that I ate while growing up. I was clueless about nutrition as a college student and during those hectic, early years as a reporter in New York and Kentucky. The lettuce and tomatoes on my fast-food burgers were vegetables enough for me.

But once I discovered the profound connection between health, healing, and nutrition, I radically changed my diet. The average person might think it's horribly strict. I mostly eat vegetables, fruits, whole grains, and lean fish. I avoid processed, fried, sugary foods. I do not ever drink any form of soda, sugar water, or alcoholic beverages. I drink only natural juices and lots of plain water.

For almost an entire decade, I consumed no red meat whatsoever. I ate only fish. Now, I incorporate organic eggs into my salads. I also use more natural supplements and vitamins.

I am very comfortable with my current diet because it is helping me feel better. I am committed to healthy eating because it one answer that I have discovered on my quest for good health. As I give my body maximum nourishment, I am working with doctors to see if the two diseases are related.

I feel confident that I'm close to answers and success. How far will I go to reach any goal I set in my life? I am always surprised at the answer to this question, but it's a simple philosophy.

As far as it takes.

Reality of Now

Journal entry: December 18, 2005

> *I don't know if, while writing a book, you're supposed to talk about writing the book. But for me, this is the perfect place to bring you into my reality of now. I took a medical leave of absence from my job in Detroit. You know, the one where I have struggled and grown. The job that I enjoy. Yep, that's the one I left.*
>
> *Now I am at a natural health institute in a beachfront community in Puerto Rico. I enter my small apartment just off the beach with more white spots than I have ever*

had. Plus, I know something more than vitiligo is making my body function improperly.

Despite this, I feel happier and more optimistic about my life than ever. Don't worry. This is not where the book turns into a mid-life crisis about a man trying to find himself. I love my job and I am going back to it in just a few months. But just about a week ago, I began to get pigment back in many white areas of my face. That's one of the most encouraging signs that I have ever had in this whole odyssey for a cure. I came here to heal myself. I know that this may be just a short period of reclamation. But I am writing down everything so that my doctors and I can understand the changes, good and bad. And find some kind of pattern or explanation in this madness.

Here they say the way to cure all ills is through diet and lifestyle. But the kicker is this: The diet consists of all raw vegan vegetarian meals and wheat grass. That means no meat, no dairy, no processed food of any kind—no exceptions. While that may sound rough, this is the place where I finally realized my change. And this change has nothing to do with any doctors, holistic healers, medications, or supplements. This big revelation has absolutely nothing to do with this place except for the peace of mind it afforded me. This place gave me the space and peace to sort through

> *my own thoughts. And in that internal journey I have*
> *made the biggest discoveries. The biggest change that I have*
> *experienced is in my mind and in my heart.*

When I sat down to write this section, I had every intention of making this part of the book about the amount and variety of healing minds I have come in contact with since I started a quest for a cure. But as this portion of the story began to take shape, the truth began to become very clear. The *cure* is not what this journey is about. This story isn't about a guy with a disease and the many different doctors he encountered—even though that is part of my journey. It's not about turning white—even though that is the reality of this disease.

It's been seven years since I won that first Emmy and decided to conquer my disease. I've spoken to doctors all over the world. Most of them were experts in their field. Many had cured people of vitiligo. Some of them I went to, some of them wouldn't even talk to me, and some of them were trying to sell me products. Since this is what some would call a cosmetic disorder, it isn't always covered by insurance. Which means I've spent thousands of my own dollars in my quest.

There are a few things I have discovered. This fact is one that was tough for me to understand: *Sometimes doctors really don't have an answer.* Even when they give you a prescription, they may make it seem like they know the diagnosis and believe that it is accurate, but they really are not sure. They are just making an educated guess and hoping they are right. Most of the time they are right. But when they are wrong, they are happy to send you to another doctor who will start the whole process all over again. I got tired of that.

So I decided to try and help. I mean I really don't expect to figure this out on my own. But the only connection between one doctor and the next sometimes is the patient. And the more information I can bring to the table the better it is for me. I began to read, research, and document my medical mission. And since then, things began to look up.

SIX

The War Within

JOURNAL ENTRY: OCTOBER 3, 2006

She kisses me on the cheek, and I begin to think. Is she OK looking into my eyes? The kisses find their way to my mouth, and now I'm focused. Her soft hands caress my face and those beautiful brown eyes lock on mine. I am there, but 100 percent of me is focused on the absolute wrong thing. You figure if she's kissing me, she has already accepted me for who I am and what I look like. But I am thinking about how she may react if she sees the rest of me. The white spots are all over my body. And I still hesitate to take off my clothes.

I am afraid. I mean, I don't think she will take off

running when I take off my shirt, but there's nothing saying she won't. The white has taken over parts of my body that I never imagined. And it would hurt if she ran off. But to be honest, it would hurt almost as much to see that hint of shock or hesitation in her eyes.

I don't want her to not want me in any way.

Maybe that's the reason I don't ever let these situations go too far. I never put myself in the situation to be disappointed … and that's why it rarely happens. But it does.

I am afraid.

I do go on dates. But they only go so far. The truth is, I don't want her to look at me funny. This is one hurdle I must conquer. I also have no desire to see my own imperfections at an intimate moment. I look at my legs or my hands, and it just reminds me of how different I am at a time I really don't want to be reminded of the situation. During a romantic moment, I should be thinking about way better stuff. But ultimately I wonder, how can this woman overlook all of this and see me for who I am and love me anyway? Because it's difficult for *me* to see me through all of this sometimes.

Most of the time, I forget I look like this. I can't see my face unless I'm in front of a mirror. And most of the time that I am at work, I'm wearing makeup. Still, even without a mirror, I am reminded of my appearance when I look at my all-white hands or take off my shirt to expose my speckled-white arms and torso. Sometimes it takes a moment, even for me, to adjust to the shocking sight of my own skin.

Suddenly I remember I'm turning white. And I don't want that moment to happen during a romantic interlude.

Still, this fear does not stop me from dating—even though I do not wear makeup when I'm off the clock. So when I ask you out and we go on a date, just know that the guy who is going to try to kiss you at the end of the night is turning white. The anxiety and anticipation for that moment has trained me to gauge how women feel about me by the time dinner is finished. If I think that she is OK with the situation, then I make my move.

I'm usually good at making the call. But sometimes, I am completely wrong. Here's one example. It was a great date. We strolled through a museum. We talked about life, love, and happiness. We had lunch at a nice restaurant downtown overlooking the river. And she seemed to be into me. I was on cloud nine. We promised to get together again in the near future. It all seemed good. Until I drove her home and pulled up in front of her building downtown. It's time for the kiss.

I express my pleasure with our outing. Then I move in for what I think will be a sure kiss. My anxiety over my appearance

121

and her reaction and potential attraction is minimal. After all, she has been looking into my face all afternoon.

I bend toward her, eager for the thrill of a goodbye kiss.

She moves away. My mind reels. We had such a great time on the date, maybe my timing or my head angle was off. You know, you don't want to bump noses. So I give it another shot. I move in for the kiss again. She moves away again, her eyes flashing with embarrassment. I'm in shock. I fumble through a confusing goodbye, then drive around the corner and sit for just a few seconds before I drive home.

How could I have let that happen? I know many guys have read a lot of signals wrong and, as a result, they get denied. But that usually happens when the girl doesn't want to see you again. Or she doesn't touch your hand while you're walking.

I know rejection is part of life. But for me, my first fear is that every time that I am rejected, it must be because of the vitiligo. I don't *know* if my look was the reason for the rejection. But every time someone treats me wrong or indifferent without reason, I automatically draw the conclusion that the shocking sight of me is what caused the mishap. It *has* to be the reason.

I don't even want to ask, because most people won't tell the truth. They don't want to say it … and I probably don't really want to hear it. In fact, I don't know what all of this means. I just know it's getting much more difficult to put myself out there.

I know I want to have love and a family. I also know that locking myself up in the house will not get me any closer to my love. But if there was ever a reason for me to hesitate to trust or put my feelings on the line, going through that kind of rejection is it.

I am afraid to try and love. But I also love everything about women. They embody the emotion, the tenderness, and seemingly everything else that we (men) are lacking.

I need them and I need love and I will never stop trying to find the right one for me. And when I do, I know that she will be someone who loves me for me.

When I connect with her, she and I will share the greatest and most rewarding love of all. And to be honest, it's the one worth waiting for. I have been rejected before and I'm sure I will be rejected again. No pain, no gain. And I can take pain if gets me closer to her.

You know ... the woman who is for me.

The Blessing of Disease

Do people see a monster or a mystery when they look at me?

I understand both reactions and make no judgments based on what I see as I figure out the answer. In all honesty, I have a mixed reaction when I see my own reflection. At my worst moments, I see a guy who screwed up so much he was punished with sickness. A disease that would not only steal love from his life, but also try to rob him of his beloved career. And it is that negative way of thinking, those doom-and-gloom thoughts, that can take over and guide a life right into the oblivion.

That way of thinking would have destroyed me. So I'm glad I kept looking. I found another view on the same reflection. Now I see beauty. I see the interesting contrast of colors. Black invaded by white in a random assault. It's shockingly interesting. And that's just on the surface. I used to hide my face and drift, with a ghost-like swiftness, through my life off camera without makeup. Now, I hold my head high with the dignified walk of a king. I am gloriously different. And this look, contrasted by the confident walk alone, is enough to make people stare.

I love the fact that my very presence can challenge people's own limitations. But most of all, I hope that it inspires them with passion just to live their best life. No matter what challenges you have, don't let anyone take your dream from you. And never give up on happiness. If you see this face of mine that gets to go on TV every day, I hope it serves as a symbol to let people know once again that there are no rules. They can accomplish anything if they just believe.

About a year ago I actually found myself with a frame of mind I would have previously never thought possible. I was thankful. Yes, thankful that I got vitiligo. Thankful that I got this disease, because it has truly brought me back to *me*. I work in a visual medium where I used to think people were judged mostly by their looks. But when my look drastically changed, I was forced to find and redefine my perception of myself. I also had to leave the possibility open that people could truly accept and love me for my inner spirit as much as for what's on the outside. And I mean a complete group of people I have never met who watch me every day on TV. I had to allow them to see me and accept me the way I am.

As I went through this transformation, I discovered that I was never satisfied with myself even before I got this disease. There was always something more I would need. Something that I just didn't have. In order to heal, I had to find out why I was never satisfied with my life before vitiligo. Another truth is that I have used vitiligo as a master excuse for not succeeding in my personal and professional lives.

"No woman could love a man who looks like this," I would tell myself. "I can't go out. People stare at me."

At the same time, I brought myself down by thinking, "*The Today Show* will never hire me."

Thankfully, I snapped out of that gloom. I can enjoy love and professional success. I reprogrammed my brain by understanding my personal history and by tweaking my current thought process accordingly.

In my quest for understanding, I spoke to my siblings, my parents, my grandmother and even some of my old girlfriends. It was a very enlightening journey. I spoke to my grandma to understand my father. I questioned my father to understand his choices in life, especially like divorce and professional struggles, the ones that affected me. I chatted with my mother with the same quest in mind. I also spoke to my sister. And even though we were in the same house and experienced the same life-changing events, her memory and my recollection of each situation were drastically different.

History is up for interpretation, I realized. I applied that epiphany to my own mind: I had the freedom and creativity to interpret and react to my experiences however I damn well pleased. I have to let go. My peace of mind depended on my ability to live, love, and let myself be loved, without holding grudges or harboring malice toward anyone.

I had to do that because my past was affecting my present. I needed to "un-learn" some of the ideas that my family had programmed into my head. They taught me everything: how to walk and talk, eat, and go to the bathroom. They shared this knowledge based on what their parents and the hard-knock life had taught them. Pile on top of that all of the biases taught about being black in America.

Having little money and an inability to express love filled

me with a sense of inadequacy. This analysis of my upbringing led me to the following conclusion: It didn't matter. My past does not define my future. Sure, all of those factors led me up to the present, but I had the power to determine my future.

I define me. I can educate myself about living better. And take the knowledge from others' struggles and use it to better my journey. That is the beautiful thing about life. At any moment you can choose to redefine yourself and actually be a better person than you were just seconds before. With every choice and every situation, you can build and get better every day—mentally and physically—freeing yourself from the constraints of your past and reprogramming yourself. The information is out there. All you have to do is find it.

I'm not saying this will be easy. The toughest person for you to change is you. The *only* person you can actually change is you. It's not easy, but once you are open to re-booting your internal programming, it can actually be fun to fight the war within.

Waging War

"The sun is not shining, so today sucks."

"My foot hurts. I must have something."

It always begins small. A couple of negative thoughts here and there. But like seeds, if you plant them in your mind, they will grow. The enemy is negative thoughts that not only can define you, but can talk you out of your dreams, your marriage, your confidence, and just about every other thing in your life. The key to having good things happen in your life is to believe that they will happen.

Damn, that seems too simple. But it's true. You also need to track your negative thoughts so you can replace them with positive ones immediately.

"It's raining outside, today sucks."

Change it to, "I should slow down today and enjoy. This is a day of growth, and water is the fuel that brings the flowers to the surface." The negative thought will come, but the more you squeeze them and replace them, the quicker they will not come at all. You also need to keep the possibility of positive things coming into your world at the forefront of your mind. The thoughts you plant in your mind are the seeds of your actions—especially your subconscious ones. The more you let thoughts linger, the more they will multiply. And whatever they are, negative or positive, they will multiply so much that they will become your truth without you even realizing it. Then you will act upon that truth.

And that's why it's important to wage war against the negative thoughts.

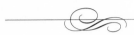

SEVEN

Public Face

I HAVE BEEN INTERVIEWING CELEBRITIES most of my professional life. And there are a few who stand out, not only for their talent, but for the way they approach life.

The biggest ones seem to have a great view on life—people like Dustin Hoffman, Meryl Streep, and Bruce Willis. But the one celebrity who has left the biggest impression on me is Will Smith. No matter if his movie is good, bad, or mediocre, he always has the most positive attitude.

I started interviewing Smith when he wasn't that famous; and his excitement, respect, and demeanor have remained genuine. During a recent interview, he said something that I'll never forget.

It happened after I asked him this question:

"I've been interviewing you since before *Independence Day* and no matter if the movie is great or bad you always have a positive attitude. How do you always maintain such a great disposition?"

Without missing a beat, he answered, "Well, that's been a lot of movies and not all of them were hits." He laughed. "To be honest with you, I fight for it. I must have positivity around me all the time. I can't work around negative energy. So if someone is around bringing the whole mood or vibe in the room down, I try to change the mood. If I can't change the mood, I will ask them to leave. And if they can't leave or I can't change the mood ... then I will go. I have to remain in a positive place for the creativity to flow. I make it a priority. I also read a lot."

Wow.

Those words have stayed with me for years. The man says he *fights* for it. He makes it a *priority*. And that explained a lot for me. This is a guy who was a big rap star and lost all of his money, only to become a star on TV and later, one of the biggest movie stars on the planet.

I like that. A priority of positivity. That is something worth fighting for.

Party Paranoia

"They call me Big L.A., Big Willie, Big Money, Big Delay."

I'm driving down the street singing, or should I say rapping, along with my favorite rapper in the world—and making up my own lyrics because I'm really not sure what he's saying. LL Cool J is the rapper and the name of the song is *Headsprung*. It's got me in the mood for a party. But something inside is trying to kill my natural high.

I'm on the way to a party at a friend's house and this is always how it begins: There's a funny feeling in my stomach that's more like moths than butterflies. This is a swank party at a well-to-do friend's house on the water. Not necessarily my crowd, but I'm daring to be different. But honestly, I don't know what to expect. I'm sure there will be some nice and interesting people. I may not know most of them but I would hope that they would be kind. At least that's always how people start out.

Then there is something in a party that always brings out the truth in a person. And that's the part of the situation that can get a little dicey for me. I understand that people will stare at me. Hell, I stare at *myself* ... but the thing that goes from people staring at me into me leaving and going home is a little social lubricant called alcohol. Drinking allows people to say what they would never say under normal circumstances. And when you see a spotted black man walk into a room you stare. As the night goes on you get more comfortable and then you may let something slip out of your mouth that has absolutely no sensitivity or empathy.

When I'm driving to any function where there will be a crowd of people I have never been around before and they will be drinking alcohol, I try to prepare myself for the worst. Too often I heard the "spotted black man" comment and the "You're almost as white as me now, man," statement.

And there's this: "My cousin has the same thing as you do, man. Here's how to fix it." Then comes the beautiful girl who walks up with a smile and that "I feel sorry for you" sympathetic look and conversation. She talks as if I'm a child, then she introduces me to everyone I just met because she feels bad for me. That sucks.

But the absolute worst is when I go to a party and everyone in the room creates one giant discussion about my disease. I'm kinda used to avoiding that, but the way my life is now, people will walk up and talk to me about it everywhere—like at the computer store or the bank.

People are inquisitive. I welcome all inquiries. Better for someone to ask than to not know. I can explain it for all of those who have this disease and can't articulate the facts. But I loathe being the vitiligo spokesman at parties! Social gatherings are supposed to be fun, relaxing, and playful, not heavy-duty discussions.

Obviously, a night out for me involves a whole lot more than choosing a venue and an outfit. Every potential dynamic of the evening plays out in my head even before I dress and while I'm driving. And if I'm the least bit reluctant to hear the worst comment, I turn around and go back home.

However, on this night, the force is with me. I refuse to allow negativity to spiral into a boring life at home watching TV. I'm heading to a gathering at a co-worker's house. I've never been there, but I feel confident that my comfort with my colleague at work will translate into comfort inside his home. While driving, I vow to remain positive and polite, no matter what anyone says.

This mental warfare is my mission for the night. It might sound like a lot of pressure. It might even strike you as crazy. But I wage this mental war every time I leave the house. Because I cannot let other people's actions or words change my mood and my world so much that I lock myself back into what I call the mental prison. That's where I imprison myself after talking myself out of going out. The crime? Fear that someone might hurt my feelings. Living this way is like never driving because you fear having an accident. That's no way to live. I have to live without worrying about feeling hurt.

Besides, hurt feelings heal, just like a small cut on your skin. Callous comments may bruise, and malicious insults may slice deep. They may even leave a scar. But they cannot cripple your passion for life. If they do, it's not the drunken guy's fault for having a loud mouth. It's yours for letting his words affect your actions. I've learned this by forcing myself to go out and face the world. Just like working out in the gym several times a week builds muscle strength, my consistent interactions with people in social settings have strengthened my positive attitude. After all, the world is mine just as much as it's the drunken guy's. And the best thing about it is that he has to share this world with me, whether he likes it or not.

A Hero Named Dustin

We are walking down the middle of Bourbon Street. And I mean the middle of the street. I'm part of a group of entertainment reporters who have come to The Big Easy to work for a couple of days. We have just seen the new film, *Runaway Jury*. And it is the night before we would interview the stars before returning home.

I had always heard of the craziness of New Orleans. People had shared their stories of wild experiences, but once I learned about the beads and the breasts, that deleted everything else from my memory. So, walking down the main street in the

French Quarter, I expected to see naked women at every turn. That didn't happen. This was pre-Katrina New Orleans— tradition and ceremony exploded around every corner. All around were people ready to tell your future, give you a riding tour, and feed you some kind of Cajun concoction. It was all there, and I was almost as excited about my visit to this city with such rich history as I was about the next day's interviews.

Runaway Jury featured Dustin Hoffman and Gene Hackman. And even though I was scheduled to get only three to four minutes with each, I was excited about the time. They are both legendary actors who have known each other since they were both struggling in New York. They are also Oscar winners.

I was very charged about the interviews. I was so gassed, I almost missed my first glimpse of the New Orleans ritual of rewarding bead-throwers with a quick flash for fun. But no one informed me that women of all ages participated in the ritual. Afterward, I went back to the hotel, disappointed but very excited about my interviews the next day.

The next morning, I walked into the hospitality suite to begin my interviewing day. I was led to believe we would get all of the principals of the film: Hackman, Hoffman, Rachel Weisz, and John Cusack. But upon my arrival, I was informed that

Gene Hackman had to leave and everyone was not going to get him. That meant I wasn't going to get to interview Hackman. So, I was a little down, but Dustin Hoffman was still on my list. And he is the one I was most looking forward to.

From *The Graduate* to *Rain Man*, Dustin Hoffman was the real deal. This was one of those times when I really loved my job.

I walked in the room ready to give my usual respectful, "How's it going? Pleasure to meet you." And I did. But as soon as I extended my hand, Hoffman looked at my hand, shook it and held on to it. He turned it over.

"Did you get a burn?" he asked.

My heart fell. I froze for a second. I had prepared myself for this moment over and over in my mind. If any of the stars I interview talk about or ask me about my hands or anything else, I would have an answer ready. You know, something snappy and amusing, such as, "I'm just disappearing slowly and color is first to go." Another one was, "Life is sucking the color right out of me."

But all of the prepared, rehearsed responses flew out of my head in that moment of silence as this Oscar winner held my hand. I remembered my personal pledge to stick with this struggle through thick and thin. But I wasn't sure if things where getting thick or not. However, I have a tried-and-true fallback plan when smooth comebacks are out the window. It's simple. Honesty. Go with the truth. At least you will escape with your dignity.

"No, it's a disease where you just start losing your pigment," I told him.

"I know how you feel," he replied. Then he lifted up his sleeves and showed me his arms. "I was burned all the way up my arms and more but most people can't see it," he confided. He showed me the burns.

"Does it work for you like it does for me?"

"What do you mean?" I asked.

"The ladies," he said. "They all want to help you and show you concern. It's a lady magnet."

I add, "Better than an Oscar." We both laugh really hard.

"We're ready," the camera crew announced. "We have speed." That means the camera is rolling and I can start my questions.

"Dustin Hoffman, it's great to sit across from you," I begin.

He answers: "I'm an African-American."

"Thank you, my brother." I give him some dat. He is familiar with the handshake and we both laugh again.

That was one of the best interviews I have ever done. And it all began with my lack of pigment.

Life is funny and Dustin Hoffman is my hero.

Momma's Boy

"I just don't want it to stop you from living your life."

This statement is among the many things my mother said to me that I will never forget. She always encouraged me to follow my dream, no matter what. And even though she could see my color continue to change, she did not want me to stop following my dreams.

Sure, it's a simple statement, but until that time, my mother and I never really spent much time talking about vitiligo. In fact, this disease just wasn't a topic of conversation with any of my family members. And to be honest with you, I don't think it should have been.

Let me explain. When I first started to lose pigment in a significant way, I went to a holistic healing center to clean out my body and learn more about healthy eating. And the people I met there were simply amazing.

My roommate was a seventy-six-year-old man who had been diagnosed with late-stage prostate cancer. His doctor had sent him home to die. But this man drastically changed his diet—and saved his life.

In fact, his doctor's death sentence had occurred fifteen years before I met the man!

Another amazing person I met at the clinic was a woman who had been diagnosed with lupus. Despite that horrifically debilitating disease, she was thriving in a way that baffled her doctor. Sadly, I also met people who were barely making it with diseases that would surely take their lives. But they were searching for hope where their doctors had given them none.

Why do I share these stories? Because meeting these people convinced me that I had no right to feel sorry for my situation. Turning white does not thrust me onto death's doorstep. The diseases that my new acquaintances were battling had the power to kill.

Vitiligo, I realized, is purely cosmetic. (I was at the clinic to find a cure for my skin condition, as I had yet to discover the cause of my back pain.) I am grateful, even jubilant, that I do not face the prospect of dying because I am turning white. I have a good job. I have a family that loves me. For goodness sake, vitiligo is not going to kill me!

Sure, I could turn white and have to check a different box on all of my personal application forms. But it will never take the most precious gift of all—my life.

So this explains why vitiligo is not a big conversation topic for me with my loved ones. My family has bigger, more important things to discuss. Things that are life-changing and perhaps even life-threatening.

In one year's time, my father had a stroke and my mother was forced to go from independent living to bed-ridden assisted living. Around the same time, one of my nephews was killed in a car accident. It seemed like we were constantly dealing with grave situations. And all these crises packed into twelve months forced my siblings and I to talk about the collective quality of life and our family's well being.

Now, we're not always in the midst of heartache. We're a family that enjoys each other's company and love to have fun as well. That's what we do. And if the subject of vitiligo does come up, it's in the context of my world. It just a small couple of sentences tucked into a talk about my entire life.

"It's getting worse, I got better makeup," I say. "Interviewed George Clooney today."

"Really? Was he cool?" And the conversation goes on.

My family and I talk about so many things it seems like we never really discussed the subject of vitiligo in depth. But we all came from the same place. And we all seemed to have a very similar view of life. My family has never even looked at me differently. When I am with them, it's like they don't even see the patches of white. Even though I know they do.

They love me without question and I them. And that way of thinking came from one place ... one person. Even though she was lying in a hospital bed at the age of seventy-four with severe rheumatoid arthritis, my mother was still worried about her baby son's life.

"Are you happy?" she would ask. "Are you healthy and eating enough?"

I think it comforted her to know that I was going to be all right, no matter what I looked like. It may be hard, but my life is good. It's funny, I don't remember everything my mother and I talked about before she died. We chatted about her childhood; I read some of her favorite books to her. We had good times, but I do remember that conversation about my well-being.

A mother's love is powerful stuff. She worried about all of her children. And even on her deathbed, she wanted to make sure I would live my best life. The way she tried to live. The way she tried to teach me.

Mom, I am and I will.

Sweet Dreams

> *I'm sitting on top of a bridge looking down over the city. It's weird because I am not scared in the least. I feel strong, invincible even. I am tough, like the guy with the paper towels that absorb everything.*
>
> *I have gone through so much and I absorb it all, never breaking, never letting anything fall through. It's cool up here. And finally I do an inventory. I see the suspension cables, the cement fortresses, and the water below. I see buildings on either side and I still don't feel afraid. I feel*

strong. I look down at my hands and see them full of color, no white at all. No patches, no nothing—and I am whole again. I keep looking around not really noticing that my hands are back to normal. I stand, reveling in my power. I jump from the bridge and begin to fly. I soar over the city—not like a bird, because I don't have to work for it. I'm a streamlined jet piercing the air. I stretch out my arms while I fly. I feel strong—ready for anything.

All of a sudden I hear the loudest horn I have ever heard. It breaks through the air faster than I can fly. Looking down, I try to find it. It's not the ship. It's not that truck. It's not coming from the warehouse on the docks. It's my alarm clock. It's time for me to get ready for work. But my dream was so vivid. The kind where you have to look around the room and take stock in reality just to make sure you were in dreamland.

It was good. I'm Brawny Thomas. And I will get up and bound to work ready to retain, flex, and stay strong and absorbent.

I laugh about the flying thing as I get to my morning ritual. I turn on the TV and watch the early news, just to make sure a major event has not changed my day. In the news business when something big happens, everyone has to report on it. I watch the network news. No big developments around the globe. I am safe to get ready for another day on television.

I sit up and still feel strong. I walk into my bathroom ready to command the shower. And it happens like it does for me at least twice a week. I catch a glimpse of myself in the mirror.

What's that on my face? I quickly look down at my hands and the rest of my vitiligo-infested body. And it hits just as hard as the first spot did when it began to claim my pigment.

I have a disease, but in my dreams I don't. And I didn't for those three minutes between my dream ending and turning the lights on, looking in the mirror, and seeing my hands.

I am dizzy with shock on mornings like when I walk into the bathroom without light, turn on those lights and recognize the reality of my world ... again.

I don't see myself like this in my mind, in my heart, and in my dreams. I see myself whole. So when I catch a glimpse of reality, it's still shocking. Very shocking. But I love the fact that when I am not conscious, I see myself complete.

I still dream and strive for what one day could be my reality. To stop dreaming even when you are awake is not good.

I maintain unwavering faith that I have a chance to get healthy. It's something to strive for while still living my life. Despite the shocking truth about my skin, it's rewarding to know that I will never change my view of me. I am happy. I am whole.

The dreams just remind me.

Show Yourself

> *"I'm Fox 2's Lee Thomas and I've interviewed some of the most famous people in the world, but there is something they never knew 'cause for years I've been covering up. Most people here at Fox 2 have never seen this. My day starts off in makeup because I think if most people saw what I look like ... they might be shocked. I'm ready to share my story."*

That was the promo commercial for a story I did about myself on TV. So it's safe to say I don't hide anymore. For the first time in my life, I gave everyone in metro Detroit a look at me without makeup on my face. The story has gotten the biggest response ever generated from any single story I have ever broadcast. Now, I wear makeup when I'm on the news simply because I think it would distract from the story if I didn't. But I only cover my face. My hands are totally white and you can see them any day you watch me on Fox 2 Detroit.

Why did I choose to reveal my disease now? One day when I was speaking to a kid on the phone—a boy who has vitiligo—he asked me to show everyone what my face looks like without the makeup. I didn't know this kid, but he had seen me at the hospital getting treatment a few years ago. First his mother called me at the station to see if I would speak to her son. She wanted me to give him some words of encouragement. He was surprised to see me on TV, with the same look that he has. I called him. He was surprised. I love kids and I love to help if I can. "It would help me if people knew your story," the young man said. So I did it.

I broadcast my face and my story all over the metro Detroit area for everyone to see, not really knowing what the response would be, but unafraid. This, from a guy who used to stay home for fear of scaring kids with his looks. Now, I was broadcasting my reality in HD where it would be available for millions to tune in. And that was the best thing I have ever done.

We received thousands of letters of support from people all over the country. Men, women, and children shared touching stories about how my journey has moved or strengthened their lives. The response was overwhelming. The joy I felt was indescribable. And now people come up to me in the street and the grocery store and everywhere else—whether I'm wearing makeup or not—and they talk with me. I love it.

But that's just the beginning. I am not only an entertainment reporter. I am now a fill-in anchor. I have actually been promoted to the desk, the job that I was once removed from (the one that sent me fleeing to the airport). Thankfully, I have overcome that obstacle as well. I feel like all of my dreams are coming true. The most incredible thing about it is that people are accepting me just as I am … white spots and all.

Right now as I write, the vitiligo is worse than it's ever been. It's not really growing much, but it's been well over a decade since I was diagnosed. It has completely whitened both hands and feet, a large part of my face and neck, and parts of my torso and legs and arms.

I'm turning white, yet I am happier than I have ever been. It's tough at times. I still struggle to go out sometimes. By the way, I've been at the station for almost a decade and my picture has never been put back on the wall. And I still have not found the woman who will share my life. But I remain hopeful.

Even with all of that in the mix, life is wonderful. I will never abandon my quest. I am still working with a doctor who is giving me some great help in managing my health and who works with me to find my way to a cure. And I am forever committed to that. If not for me, then for the child that I hope to have one day. The theories on this disease are just theories. I know that some say this is genetic and some say it's not. Whichever the case, I don't want the child I one day wish to father to deal with this … ever.

When I started writing this book, I wanted to end it with the declaration, "I found a cure!" I envisioned a picture of myself on the back cover, grinning from a face that had re-pigmented and resumed its natural brown color. How could I end this any other way? But this ending is much more appropriate. Yes, I am a black man with a disease. It seems beyond my control. But I'm still fighting. And even though this is part of my journey in life, it is not the whole story of me. I will not let it be. I will not let it control or define me. If I quit and go hide somewhere, I will have truly lost. The disease would have taken complete control of the direction of my life. Vitiligo would have won.

Winning for me is just staying in the game. It's simply about getting up and showing up. Showing up at work, at parties, on dates, and everywhere else life takes me. It's simply about making sure I can live the life that I want to live.

I can continue to do the job that I worked hard to secure. No matter what anyone says.

Teenagers may still laugh and call me chocolate and vanilla, like at the mall the other day. I like ice cream.

I had a celebrity recently refuse to shake my hand; said he had a cold. I understand. But if I shake every celebrity's hand in Hollywood or if I become the poster boy for chocolate/vanilla swirl, certain things will never change. I am Lee Willie Thomas Jr.—loving son, brother, and uncle. I make my living as an award-winning reporter who has been promoted to news anchor. I love people, especially kids, and one day I will have a family of my own. I am extremely happy and proud of my life, and I will try with each moment to be a better person than I was the moment before.

The key for me is simple: *Just live!* Keep showing up and continue to engage life. We need each other to survive. I will never give up on loving life or sharing it with people. And no person or thing can change any of that.

Even if I am turning white.

Acknowledgements

I DIDN'T THINK MY STORY WAS THAT UNIQUE until I had a telephone conversation with a young man who had vitiligo. This young man shared the story of an even younger boy he knows who wears a mask because he's afraid to show his face.

In telling me about their struggles, he made things very clear for me. He said with media exposure maybe people would see *my* story and treat *him* differently. He went on to say if I just explained the disease, maybe things could change for people struggling to deal with vitiligo.

I would like to thank him for his insight. And for inspiring me to tell my story.

The majority of this book is taken from my journals;

some quotes and descriptions came from taped interviews. My written notes are not as extensive as I would like, and memory is fallible, but there are no made-up characters or situations. Names were left out, but everyone is real. Also, the vitiligo information is from the National Vitiligo Foundation. (See *Resources*, page 152.)

I also need to acknowledge Beverly Golston, Rena Randall, Mike Thomas, Russell Thomas, and the rest of my family for accepting me no matter what.

My colleague, photographer Mike Shore, found the drama, beauty, and reality of the disease's progression and documented the changes with multiple photo shoots over the course of four years. Thank you for making it OK for people to stare. And to his wife Amy for her continuing support.

Thank you Elizabeth Atkins, writer of ten books. Your advice helped me to communicate from the heart, and you are a constant inspiration. Juan Lee has always been an angel on my shoulder. Alicia Dean for her constant input, patience, and undying encouragement. Thank you Dr. Lim and Henry Ford Multicultural Dermatology Center in Detroit for creating a place beyond medicine where vitiligo patients can find emotional support.

Thanks to my bosses, Dana Hahn and Jeff Murri, along with all of my colleagues at WJBK Fox 2 Detroit. After a decade with you it is more than a job, it is a home. Thank you for the freedom to be me.

To Ed Peabody, Steve Wilke, and the team at Momentum Books, thank you for your expertise, professionalism, and personal touch.

And last but definitely not least, to the hundreds of thousands of viewers in the metro Detroit area, my look changed and you still watched. Thank you for allowing me into your homes. And even more than that, thank you for allowing me the privilege of telling your stories. We have shared life and I love you for that. I may have been born somewhere else, but like some of the best cars in the world, I was made in Detroit.

Thank you all.

Lee Thomas,
September 2007

Resources

National Vitiligo Foundation
WWW.NVFI.ORG

WJBK Fox 2 Detroit
WWW.MYFOXDETROIT.COM

Turning White Foundation
WWW.TURNINGWHITE.COM

Optimum Health Institute
WWW.OPTIMUMHEALTH.ORG

Vitiligo Support International
WWW.VITILIGOSUPPORT.ORG